BEHIND THE WHITE COAT

INTIMATE REFLECTIONS ON BEING A DOCTOR IN TODAY'S WORLD

ISBN 0-9724261-0-8

Published 2002

Published by Steven H. Farber, 103 Wind Ridge Circle, The Woodlands, TX 77381, U.S.A.

Printed in Canada

Cover and Interior Design: Andra Keller
Front Cover photo: Corbis
Back Cover photo: Roger Fowler
Illustrator: GS Davis

BEHIND THE WHITE COAT

INTIMATE REFLECTIONS ON BEING A DOCTOR IN TODAY'S WORLD

Steven H. Farber, M.D., F.A.C.C.

To those who have healed me with their love

&

To those whom I have lovingly tried to heal

Acknowledgments

I would like to express sincere gratitude to Celia Rocks, my publicist, for believing in my work when others didn't. I would like to express special appreciation to Angela Adair-Hoy of Booklocker for her assistance; the members of the Woodlands Writers Guild for their constructive criticism and support; Tracy Welch and Mike Davis for their editorial help and encouragement; Valerie Ott, Christie Rogers, and Rachel Feeler for helping me with their computer skills to organize my book; my wife, Beverly, for her love and support in spite of numerous hours away from both my family and from the work that I needed to do around the house; my children, who I hope will always remember that the most important initials after my name stand for "My Daddy"; my mother and late father for supporting me through my struggles to become a doctor while they themselves struggled; my sister Harriet, for being there when I have needed her; and finally my precious Muse for giving me constant inspiration that touched the depths of my soul in a way that it had never been touched before.

Table of Contents

Introduction

A Blessing and a Curse

Like many young doctors, I was naïve and foolish enough to think that I had the world by the tail. I had graduated from both college and medical school with honors, and at the age of twenty-six, I thought that I was smart enough to figure out the answers to all of life's problems. After four rugged years of training, I was embarking on a world that was even more exciting and demanding, the world of residency training at the renowned Baylor College of Medicine. Little did I know "how much I didn't know" or understand about the system that we call "modern medicine."

My ancestors had struggled to come to America from a foreign land, and I was proud to be the first doctor in my family. Youthful idealism filled my being, and like many idealists, material goals were not my primary objective nor money my main concern. After all, doctors perform great and miraculous things; Michael DeBakey, Denton Cooley, and Christiaan Barnard were all my childhood heroes. They were among the people that I admired and looked up to; they represented the nobleness and goodness that life had to offer.

In my youth, most books that I read glorified doctors, making them almost superhuman. Denton Cooley was my "Mickey Mantle of Medicine," and since I am a die-hard Yankee fan, that was no small accomplishment! The heroes of medicine had totally seduced me with their awesome power to control life and death and to hold people's fates and futures in the palms of their hands. My own idealism and medicine's heavy-hitters had won me over.

Years later, I have a very different vision of medicine and a more experienced view of life in general, one that is less glamorous and more realistic. Being a doctor has been a two-edged sword, and I was ill equipped and unprepared to handle it without cutting myself and suffering the consequences of my ignorance.

Medicine has opened many doors for me, but there was no way of knowing what was on the other side, or that it might hit me in the rear as I walked through. There were no instruction books about how to live a doctor's life or about what to expect when I finished my education.

Medical training teaches many invaluable lessons but nothing about life or about the "real world." I had no way of imagining the struggles that were ahead of me. The obstacles that faced me personally and professionally were things that would have been nightmares had they been dreams. Like most doctors, my training taught me how to pass tests but taught me nothing about how to "pass life."

While this book is about the experiences and journey of one doctor, I want to dispel popular myths while shedding light on a "human side" that most of the public has no way of understanding. I want to share with you the perils and frustrations that doctors face every day of their professional lives.

In order to do this, I am going to tell you a lot about myself. This is a candid story of what it is like to both become a doctor and to live the life that comes with the title. Most of what I learned came after the initials "M.D." were added to my name.

It is true that many of life's lessons cannot be learned from textbooks or a formal curriculum but can only be extracted from living. My life as a doctor has been no exception. I hope that this book will give you some insights into the life of a doctor by giving you the benefit of my experiences, both good and bad. My fervent hope is that understanding my life will teach you something that may benefit you or someone close to you.

Beauty and passion are part of the daily life of a doctor, but, unfortunately, so are the sights of suffering, pain, and death. These elements have a huge impact on a doctor's emotional makeup. Although we can never become immune to suffering, there are ways of coping with internal pain that will help us heal our own wounds and more effectively soothe the pain of others.

You are going to read about a nemesis that has plagued the medical profession—managed care—and how it affects a doctor's relationship with his patients. You are also going to hear what may be a different viewpoint about malpractice and how our legal system affects the costs and quality of medical care. It is important for all of us to understand that there is a humorous side to both medicine and to life and that it is important to be able to laugh at life's absurdities and to laugh at our own mistakes.

A doctor's life is both a blessing and a curse. The blessing is the pleasure and satisfaction of helping others improve the quality of their lives; the curse is that medicine, through the intense self-sacrifice that it requires, leaves a doctor prone to physical and emotional illness. The process of creating doctors produces well-educated, but sometimes sick, physicians who are sent out into the world to heal others.

I want you to understand that the life of a doctor is a story of an agony and an ecstasy that can take you to the deepest of valleys and help you ascend to the highest of mountaintops. There are days when the fatigue and stress are so unbearable that I curse my decision to ever don a white coat and wear a stethoscope. There are also times when being a doctor allows me to feel a "high" so intense that it could only be compared to the miracle of childbirth.

Self-esteem and peace of mind can't be achieved by merely donning a white coat or by applying makeup to improve the reflections in our mirrors. Our true value as human beings is found not only within our minds and hearts but also in the spiritual and human relationships that define our characters. Our feelings of self-worth must reside in something far greater than "what" we are; it is "who" we are that is vitally important.

Physicians are not healers by virtue of their titles. They must have something far greater than fancy diplomas, prestige, and a bunch of initials after their names. Hopefully, by telling my own tale, I can show you that being a doctor is entirely about being human.

You are about to read about my hidden battles, bitter disappointments, frustrations, and personal victories. The ensuing pages describe some of the most vivid and intense memories of the life of a doctor. I want you to understand more about the person *Behind the White Coat.*

I hope that, if you are a young doctor, you can avoid the pitfalls that I fell into while enjoying opportunities and an excitement that no other career can offer. This book is not meant to discourage you but instead give you the benefits of my years of experience and allow you to go into medicine with your eyes wide open. Those who are acquainted with doctors will obtain a better understanding of their friends, neighbors, and relatives.

Patients need to understand their rights and the impact that the wonderful yet often frustrating world of medicine has on their care. They need to face the realities of our system with awareness instead of ignorance. This book is dedicated to both doctors and their patients.

Chapter 1

Indoctrinating a Doctor

Choices

Of all the phrases that define medical school and internship training, "sink or swim" and "trial by fire" are the most synonymous with the educational process that is used to prepare young physicians to go out into the world of modern medicine. This process, in a real sense, is an indoctrination and starts early in college where grades and high scores count for everything. Many classes are cutthroat, where success requires an A or a B at the very least; and students know that only a precious few are allowed passage into the next stage of medical training. Some would do most anything to succeed.

During my freshman year of college, I spent long hours studying while others were going to parties and mixers. Like most pre-meds, I initially majored in biology. Biology majors ate, slept, and studied to beat the fierce competition. All-nighters were not uncommon before big exams. Long hours of required studying were meant to prepare future doctors not only for the rigors of medical school and the life that followed, but it was also a way of weeding out those who couldn't hack it or just didn't want it badly enough.

It didn't take long for me to realize that all-nighters and I didn't agree with each other. I didn't sleep at all the night before my first big exam because I wanted to get the best score possible. Besides, all the other Bio Sci (Biological Sciences) majors were doing it; it was necessary to keep up with the competition. Students were up in the wee hours of the morning cramming every fact that they could into every last exhausted synapse of their brains.

I got a "D" on my first exam because I was so tired that I couldn't think straight. "To hell with this!" I vowed to get to bed at 10 P.M. and get a decent night's sleep prior to the remainder of the exams. My friends were incredulous about my newly discovered work ethic. I aced the remainder of the exams and felt better physically and mentally.

The most important lesson that I learned during my freshman year of college was that I functioned better with a decent night's sleep. "All-nighters" would best be left to the cutthroats, who would probably sell their souls for a good grade.

Sometime during my freshman year, I discovered that I felt unhappy and out of place in the midst of this endless stream of pressure. Nightmares and panic attacks awakened me the night before big exams, and I felt uncomfortable with the backstabbing that seemed to go along with being a pre-med. My personality just didn't fit into the mold that I had poured myself into and that had become my life.

Feeling discouraged, I met with my advisor and asked for his advice. All pre-meds have faculty advisors. After listening to the speech I had prepared, he informed me that if I switched my major, my chances of getting into med school would be virtually nonexistent. He advised me to deal the best that I could with the situation. The hardships were only temporary. After all, I had to prove that I could handle the pressure of being a Biology major if I wanted to be accepted into medical school. "The sacrifice is worth it," he said. "Being an English major is for sissies."

Self-sacrifice became my modus operandi at the age of eighteen. It became the code to live by.

After quite a bit of soul-searching, I decided to be "a sissy" and not heed his advice. I adopted English as my major. Unsure of what I wanted in life, I decided to take the prerequisites to get into medical school without being a traditional biology major.

My advisor shook his head in disapproval and disbelief at the news, and like a stern father, he warned, "You'll never get into medical school. You might as well forget about it." I'll never forget his words because I wanted him to eat them so badly. At the time, I was an impressionable freshman, and he shook my confidence. But my competitive instincts were intact, and I held steadfast to my choice by remembering "***Me.***"

Choices

Choices are often not easy,
Tho' at times we make them harder
Than they need to be,
By forgetting to please "me."

Pleasing "me" is a must
Like eating or tying your shoe,
Why do we forget to trust
"me," to tell us what to do?

In retrospect, I made the only choice that I could, a choice that was necessary to preserve my sanity and survival. A world was also opening to me that would give me an opportunity to study a variety of literary works and to read things that would never cross my path again. My senior honors thesis was based upon a Freudian interpretation of *Othello*. I was busy dissecting Shakespeare instead of cats and dogs, and I was enjoying it.

There was something about my professors that fascinated me. Back in the sixties, long hair and baggy jeans were commonplace among liberal arts teachers. Biology professors never seemed to want to sit back and contemplate the world. They were too busy driving in the fast lane to God knows where. They dressed and acted like "the establishment," which was a popular term at the time.

English professors were laid back and discussed the future of mankind and important philosophical issues. They were a liberal breed and had a different way of thinking from what I was accustomed to. They specialized in dissecting thoughts instead of animals. It presented a unique challenge and a different set of difficulties.

I remember tasting a sense of freedom when our campus went on strike during the spring of 1970 when the United States bombed Cambodia. At long last, I was expressing myself and making my own decisions. In reality, I was following the crowd. It was in vogue to dislike Richard Nixon and distrust the government if you lived on a college campus in the late sixties.

It is important to do well on the MCATS (medical school aptitude tests) and have a high grade point average to be accepted into medical school. Fortunately, I was able to do both and was accepted by three schools.

Some of my science-oriented buddies argued that I got into medical school through the back door. That didn't bother me too much; I had worked hard to finally achieve my goal, and I felt incredible satisfaction when I got there.

Besides, being an English major gave me the time to decide what I wanted to do with my life (which was not until my junior year) and not get caught up in the inertia of a pre-med program. Instead, I tried my best to emulate my English professors and found myself puffing on pipes and trying to sound scholarly. I read Shakespeare by day and dissected frogs by night.

I really don't know if people are happier or better off if they read Shakespeare. However, having something in my life that is distinctly non-medical has proven to be an important stress-relieving outlet and an escape valve when the pressure has gotten too tough to handle. My patients have indirectly benefited from Shakespeare even if they didn't know who he was or couldn't afford to see his plays.

An obvious corollary to having been an English major is that I can now look at life in terms of drama. My "to be or not to be" turned into the "slings and arrows of outrageous fortune" within a matter of a few years. Unfortunately, some of those arrows wound up being aimed at me. As you will soon find out, my life would have made good subject matter for a Shakespearean play, one that could be called *A Comedy of Errors*.

Around that time, medical schools started to adopt the philosophy that it is important for doctors to be well rounded. A thorough knowledge of science is not enough; it is important to know something about the humanities in order to take care of human beings. It made perfect sense to me.

College gave me my first experiences with the pressure that accompanies medical training. It is important to understand that a lot of this pressure is directed from within. Many doctors are compulsive people by nature and have a hard time not being uptight. They tend to be perfectionists and have chosen a field that requires a high standard of excellence from themselves and from others. In my case, I became a perfectionist at an early age. This trait caused me a lot of frustration. The problem was that I didn't realize how hard it is to be perfect in an imperfect world.

Some of us are poured into a mold to succeed from the time we are born. I was the grandson of immigrants, and education was a top priority for my family. Sports were not discouraged but definitely ranked second to academics. I loved sports, but although I had a lot of heart and enthusiasm, I had very little talent. My physical abilities were proof that "white boys can't jump." I had to move my dreams into a different arena, away from "jocks" and into the world of needles and syringes. What a drop in income and prestige!

I was highly motivated by a strong sibling rivalry with a sister four years older than me who was extremely successful. I was bred with a competitive fire from an early age, and I knew that I had to follow in her footsteps. It was expected, and it was a birthright; there were no alternatives. Failure was not an option. Success was a way of life in my family. I came to need it, and at the same time, I hated the pressures that it represented; it was a love-hate relationship.

My ancestors carried a heavy load on their shoulders when they came to Ellis Island and Galveston almost a century ago. They wanted me to have a better life than the one they had known, and they knew that opportunity came with education, as well as with courage and hard work.

My grandparents' net worth consisted primarily of intangibles such as hard work and integrity. Frivolities were unheard of and self-indulgence a rarity. Eating out, which more recent generations take for granted, was considered a luxury and a waste of money. My grandparents fought over who was going to prepare the next meal.

Grandpa Sol, or "Gegi" (short for the Yiddish term "shmagegi"), usually got his way in what was a male-dominated world. Survival required a strict code of conduct. This was manifested in many aspects of their lives, in their spiritual beliefs, their work ethic, their financial decisions, and their morality.

It is true that the apple doesn't fall far from the tree. My grandparents' beliefs were passed on, in turn, to my parents. My father was a high school teacher and guidance counselor. He was compassionate but very demanding. He expected me to work hard, and he supported me not just with money but also with his guidance and love.

My mother was a secretary for the board of education. She, along with my dad, made education a top priority in my life. It was a must! My mother taught me a lot about how to treat people fairly and with compassion. Neither pressured me to become a doctor, but they were willing to sacrifice material things to help me get there. After all they had done, I couldn't bungle the job.

A lot of people are not descendants of immigrants, but they carry the same desire, work ethic, and need to succeed. Doctors make a conscious decision to go into a profession that is physically and mentally one of the most grueling and demanding professions that ever existed. It has to fit your nature like a suit is tailored to fit your body. Becoming a doctor fulfilled my goal of becoming a success, but I had no idea that "The Oath of Hippocrates" meant more than a pretty diploma hanging on the wall.

Medical school was tough but was made bearable by the fact that I was graded on a pass/fail system. That may scare some of you who want to know if your doctor graduated first or last in his class. To be honest, I passed with honors, but after four years of what I could only describe as pure purgatory, I didn't care if it was by one point or by fifty. When it came to surviving medical school, I was just happy to pass and graduate. Only the most compulsive among us wanted to know if they had done a better job passing than everyone else. I felt sorry for those who took life too seriously.

Medical school was also my first, and, unfortunately, not my last, experience with losing a friend to suicide. No one among us ever knew why Fred ended his life. He had injected himself with morphine that he had taken from the hospital, jumped out of his dormitory window, and was found the next morning. We all were terribly distraught and perplexed. Fred was a fallen comrade, a fellow with whom we had gone into battle; and his action made us stop to think about our own mortality and vulnerability.

Friends with "Frankie"

Medical school taught me a lot about death, and it did it by force-feeding it to me on a daily basis. My classmates and I dissected our cadavers for a ten-month period that seemed more like an eternity; bit by bit I cut into every part of his cold flesh until it no longer resembled anything human. I spent long hours with an alcoholic who died of cirrhosis in a lonely room filled with fifty other people, all of who were dead except for me. It sounds crazy, but my cadaver and I became buddies. I even nicknamed him "Frankie," short for Frankenstein.

My pre-exam routine was to study in the anatomy lab until midnight and grab a bite to eat at the café a block from the school in downtown Philadelphia. My hands often smelled like formaldehyde, but my hunger overpowered the stench because I hadn't had time for dinner, and I would usually be ravenous. My friends would sometimes meet me, and we would swap tales about our cadavers. We had to see who had the funniest anatomy lab jokes and the craziest stories and experiences.

The smells that I took home on my body and clothing were surreal and grotesque. They permeated my daily existence; they would have made life unbearable if I hadn't found ways to tolerate their presence. The smells were there no matter how hard I washed my hands. They were embedded in my hair, my clothes, my skin, and in the innermost recesses of my mind.

On the way home, walking down Broad Street, I would look at the homeless people sitting or lying on the sidewalks or storefronts and wonder who would be under the scalpel of next year's medical student rookies. Unfortunately, this was the destiny of many of these poor people before they became unwilling participants in some medical school curriculum. I felt sorry for them and considered myself lucky to be on the other side of the scalpel.

Those long hours also taught me how to distance myself from death. When I was young, the fear of death was overpowering. Nightmares clouded the death of friends and loved ones, and I didn't want to be around something so hideous and appalling. Somehow, I had to find a way to cope with my fears. There was no choice but to learn to tolerate death's inevitability in order to survive. At the same time, I had to somehow figure a way to detach myself from it in order to keep my sanity.

I didn't realize until much later that I had not yet come to terms with my own mortality. Death created pain, and the way to deal with pain was to distance myself from its source. The art of distancing was something that I would use later over and over again to defend myself from anything that could hurt me. A lot of Fred's friends distanced themselves from the events surrounding his death; it was the easy way out.

Thus, death became just another hurdle in life that had to be conquered. After all, wasn't I becoming a doctor in order to delay, defeat, or even cheat death? Learning how to fight death gave me, at the time, a sense of power that camouflaged my lack of understanding. I didn't realize until later that death was sometimes a welcome friend, and at times, it was an event that was prayed for. For some, it was a blessing and a release from pain and suffering.

On Top of Mount Everest

It took willpower and determination to make it through all the tough times in medical school. After what seemed like an eternity, my class graduated, and we received our diplomas and the initials that we had yearned for. I was neither the best nor the worst in my class, but I could have cared less. I graduated with honors and was elected to Alpha Omega Alpha, the national medical honor society. But to be honest, I was thankful to have survived.

At my graduation, my family was beaming with pride, and my classmates and I felt almost a sense of exhilaration from the success that we had achieved. I felt like Sir Edmund Hillary after he had conquered Mt. Everest. We were a group of young doctors who felt ready to conquer the evil forces of illness with all the strength that we could muster. We had captured our dreams and had not succumbed to the intense pressure. The worst certainly was behind us, or so we thought.

There was a slight miscalculation: we had no idea what was in store for us. Lives that had so neatly fit into so many categories and that had been based on success algorithms were about to meet the toughest challenges of them all. We were about to be thrown into the vivid reality of patient care and pressures of an entirely different kind.

The First Date

There are certain red-letter days in a person's life that are unforgettable because they help to define the very essence of that human being. For a doctor, one such day is the day that he dons his white coat for the first time and carries his stethoscope and little black bag into a patient's room and takes a history and physical examination on a real live human being!

The "little black bag" and stethoscope are the basic required hardware, and they are given to a medical student early in his career. I remember looking at them longingly, wondering when I would get the opportunity to put all those years of classroom work into action.

Medical school generally requires two years of classroom work followed by two years of clinical training on the wards of an affiliated teaching hospital. Hahnemann was a little different and alternated years; the first year was academic, the second year clinical, etc. Most of us were excited to be able to start seeing patients and having "hands-on" experience, and we couldn't wait. This was what it was all about!

The day that I examined my first patient was September 12, 1974. I felt as scared and excited as when I was preparing to go out on my first date with a girl, which was some seven years earlier. Trembling, I donned my white coat and took my little black bag filled with the traditional accoutrements onto the hospital ward. Sweat poured off my brow, and beads of perspiration dotted my shirt. Inside, I was shaking.

I entered the patient's room like a soldier preparing to go into battle. I tried to hide my nervousness behind a façade of calm confidence. Surely, I didn't want this little elderly woman to know that I was a "virgin" doctor and that she was my first patient. Later, I realized that she probably saw through me.

Medical students are taught to take thorough history and physical examinations. This sometimes takes hours and requires page after page of writing, especially in the beginning. Taking a good "H and P" is an art, and it is an essential part of becoming a doctor. Over time, you learn to be concise. In the beginning, nothing could be left out, and that meant that medical students had to get over their fear of doing exams on very private parts of the anatomy. It also meant that you had to become comfortable discussing some very personal subjects with people who are total strangers.

My patient was an elderly woman in her seventies. She had emphysema and was admitted to the hospital with shortness of breath. Calmly and politely, she sat with me and answered my questions. The question-and-answer period took about an hour because the "review of systems" covers a wide range of material about each organ system. Many of these subjects had nothing to do with her illness, but nothing could be omitted.

Finally, the time came for me to perform the physical examination. Medical students are taught to start at the head and to "work your way down" to the feet. The *piece de resistance* came at the very end and consisted of a rectal exam and pelvic for women and a rectal and genital exam for men. Ouch! That was the part that I really dreaded! My practice runs had taught me that in certain instances, giving is not always better than receiving.

My elderly little patient, whom I had gotten to know so well over the preceding hour, finally broke the ice in a way that I could never have predicted. I took out my ophthalmoscope, which is an instrument used for examination of the "eye grounds" or retinas, and started my eye examination. This procedure requires being nose to nose with the patient, which is sometimes quite an uncomfortable position.

About a minute or two into the examination, she said to me, "Doctor, I haven't been this close to a man in years!" We both shared the moment with laughter. In that instant, she helped me to get over my nervous jitters, and I was able to finish the examination without the tension that I had initially felt.

On the way out the door, I commented with a sigh, "I think you look pretty good."

She replied, "I think you do too!"

I was thankful to her for being gentle with her young inexperienced doctor. I'll never forget her for as long as I live. She did me a huge favor at a time when I needed one.

The Philosophy of "See One, Do One, Teach One"

Medical school is a young doctor's first exposure to the time-honored tradition of "see one, do one, teach one." When I first heard this expression, I thought it was just a joke; but when the time came for me to start my first intravenous line and stick a needle into the vein of another human being, I realized that it was stark reality. Drawing blood from another human being for the first time is an unforgettable experience for a young doctor.

First, an intern-teacher showed us how to properly cleanse an area of skin with an alcohol-soaked cotton ball. He then proceeded to carefully insert a needle into a patient's vein. We were asked to practice on each other and then repeat the same procedure on our assigned patients. My hand trembled as I carefully guided the needle towards its target. A fellow medical student made a good test subject. I hit pay dirt on the first try! My eyes were closed, and I prayed as he guided a needle back in my direction. Luckily, he was successful, and he didn't have to twist and turn the needle to find the excellent veins in my arm.

The next targets were our patients. They were not quite as fortunate as we were because their veins were more hidden and damaged from illness and also from having been "stuck" on numerous occasions. My first attempt was a miss; it took several punctures to find my mark. Fortunately, the subject of my efforts was sedated, on a ventilator, and didn't feel a thing. I didn't want to hurt him while I took target practice.

Other procedures were taught and learned in a similar manner. I saw one arterial stick, one bone marrow, and one (or if I was lucky, two) of most everything else. Wearily, I went about trying to emulate my teachers. My unfortunate patient-victims were sometimes stuck as many as ten times in the very beginning before I learned my way around a needle.

Asking for help was done only as a last resort. It was basically admitting defeat, which is hard for most medical students to do. None of us wanted to be the one who didn't have the "right stuff." Our evaluations also depended on our abilities to get the job done. In the meantime, I prayed that my patients would be sedated enough to be unaware of my fervent and often futile efforts.

It took awhile, but I eventually adopted the philosophy of "three strikes and I'm out." Now if I can't accomplish my goal in three attempts, I yell for help. The problem is that someone else is not always available to bail you out of trouble, and you often have no choice but to do the best you can when you are alone, especially in the middle of the night.

But when you are tired and frustrated, a fresh look from someone else is necessary for your patient's sake. Sometimes admitting defeat is the compassionate and humane way to treat both yourself and your patient. Unfortunately, compassion sometimes took a back seat to my need for a good evaluation and my basic instincts for survival. My foolish pride and fears of failure sometimes got in the way of seeking help when I should have.

Luckily, over time, I became very adept at finding blood vessels and began to enjoy the challenge. I also became less concerned about asking for help. There were also, however, times when patients actually became targets for venting my anger and frustration, and the "three-strike rule" didn't apply.

Sometimes, I found myself muttering in the back of my tired mind, "How dare you get sick and deprive me of sleep? You'll pay the price with this dull, dirty needle!" Of course, the needle was never dull or dirty, but sometimes I felt better if I imagined that it was!

The philosophy of "see one, do one, teach one" doesn't apply to major surgery. But this method of teaching has been handed down from generation to generation of doctors, perhaps under a different name. For better or for worse, it is part of the "basic training" of our young doctors.

Often, understandably frustrated nurses who assisted us with our procedures could be heard grumbling, "God save us, here comes another medical student with a needle…run and hide!"

They scattered in all directions when they saw the frightened student or intern approach with the "deer in the headlight" look on his face. I couldn't blame those nurses; a lot of us were pretty inept in the beginning, and they were afraid for their patients. Fortunately, most of us became better with lots of practice. Some just took more time to get there. But just how do doctors "practice" medicine?

"Practicing" Medicine

After medical school, I needed a change of scenery. The home of DeBakey and Cooley in Houston, Texas, seemed like a logical choice to propel me into the arena of modern medicine. What better training could a young doctor receive than with the revered modern patriarchs of American medicine, the icons of millions throughout the world? Fantastic, mind-boggling medical events routinely came out of Houston, Texas. The Texas Medical Center with its skilled heart surgeons was famous worldwide. Baylor College of Medicine offered the prestige that fed my ego. It was enough of an aphrodisiac to entice me to travel halfway across the country in a small car with my belongings in my U-Haul™ and my cat in the back seat.

It didn't take long for me to realize that I was about to face the greatest challenge of my young life. There was a vast difference between medical school and internship versus residency training. My senior year of medical school had given me only a limited taste of what was to come. Fledgling doctors can't fathom how their fantasies will yield to the harsh stark reality of the real world. "Boot camp" was about to begin!

New medical school grads start out as **houseofficers** who are expected to take a larger and more responsible role in patient care. It is not unusual to find yourself up at all hours of the night sticking people with needles; getting stool, urine, and sputum specimens; even performing a lot of the tests yourself in the laboratory. I had difficulty getting used to the smells of feces and vomit. They made me retch and feel faint. I often wondered whether my stomach was strong enough to withstand the odors and sights of medicine. Maybe being smart just wasn't enough? A cast-iron stomach would have been a great help. Others seemed unfazed by things that had me clinging to the commode.

Interns have to learn to budget their time; sometimes this meant taking patients back and forth to the x-ray department so that tests would be done before morning report and rounds. Reports had to be back quickly, and being fast and efficient was not only essential, but it was also part of survival. You learned to be fast if you wanted to sleep and eat. Any extra time beyond that was a luxury.

When I was an intern, support services at the indigent care facilities were thin, and the **housestaff** often filled in the huge gaps. On the other hand, in the private hospitals, there were more nurses, lab technicians, and transport personnel. These support services made life a lot easier because they allowed doctors to get some sleep. The housestaff could count on others to get the job done instead of having to do everything themselves. The Baylor program included Ben Taub, a large indigent-care facility supported with public funds, the VA Hospital, the Methodist, and St. Luke's, the last two being large, privately owned facilities.

For those of you without a medical background, I need to explain some basic definitions. Housestaff consists of **interns** and **residents** who are in a strict pecking order, the intern being lowest, and the senior resident being the highest on the ladder. The **scut** work is the busy work that no one else wants to do and consists of things such as getting lab reports and drawing blood. Senior residents are generally allowed as much sleep as possible because they have already paid their dues; it is a matter of respect. Also, they have the responsibility of supervising the interns and first-year residents.

The housestaff becomes a team and the senior resident, its leader. We made sure that lab reports and treatment plans were on the patients' charts by morning report, which is the presentation of cases by the housestaff to the faculty about each of the patients that had been admitted over the past day.

The intern has the responsibility of seeing that all the necessary tests are ordered and that the results are charted before 7 A.M.; this includes a detailed history and physical, progress notes, and treatment plan. The charting alone could take hours, and it was unacceptable for charts to be incomplete at morning report, which resembled a chart audit. That feat usually translated into getting little or no sleep and going to morning report loaded with caffeine and feeling exhausted and haggard. My memories went back to my early days in college when I tried to pull all-nighters and couldn't function well the next day; my body still rebelled intensely. Unfortunately, it never got better with time. People who said that I would get used to it were wrong.

The intern is the first in the line of fire, being the apprentice of the upper-level residents. Then comes the **attending physician,** the faculty member in charge of the ward. His job is to teach the housestaff about their cases and to make sure they practice good, sound, and safe medicine. He is "The Commanding General." "Patton," as some of us called our attending, fired questions at the intern after he or she presented the case. A differential diagnosis was expected, which meant a list of the possible diseases that could best explain the patient's symptoms and physical findings.

Unfortunately, at these rounds, teaching often became somewhat of an inquisition. My fellow interns, exhausted and hyped up on caffeine, did their best to answer difficult medical questions about their patients. Last-second reading was squeezed in between a quick shower and a cup of coffee before morning report in an attempt to bone up on the anticipated questions.

The attending and senior residents, usually more rested and on their toes, contrasted with the pathetic, disheveled figures in front of them. Many of the senior residents could sympathize with the intern who stumbles into the room, hair unkempt, and eyes puffy and bloodshot. That's because they, too, had been interns a few years earlier. Morning report was essentially trial by fire with the interns almost literally walking on coals. The teaching process was also a form of hazing, and the playing surface wasn't even.

On one occasion—after having been up all night in the ICU, or Intensive Care Unit, taking care of a critically ill patient—my attending grilled me mercilessly during the morning report. Unfortunately, I had had little time to do extra reading or prepare myself for his questions, and I answered them poorly.

Mentally exhausted from my difficult night, I felt humiliated in front of my fellow interns and residents. I ran from the room in tears, thinking that maybe I just was not tough enough or smart enough to become a doctor. Exhaustion had left me totally drained, and I had nothing left to give. Luckily, I made it through the rotation, but I doubted my abilities for the first time and wondered whether I had what it takes.

Internship is filled with extended periods without sleep, often for thirty-six hour stretches, sometimes longer. I went extended periods without a day off, working twelve-hour shifts for a solid month in the Ben Taub Emergency Room (E.R.), a place filled with enough pathology and carnage to fill a medical textbook or a horror flick. My daily routine was to work, stumble home (often seeing double because my eyes were tired during the drive), grab a few hours of sleep, eat a bite, and return for the next twelve hours. In between I tried to spend time with friends, but the schedule just didn't allow too much socializing. You had to eat, sleep, and conserve your energy as much as possible because you were back on the merry-go-round the next morning, but I'll talk more about the E.R. in a few minutes.

I made mistakes from exhaustion, mistakes that caused me to be a less efficient doctor and, at times, possibly even dangerous. I remember thinking to myself that only a superman could work these kinds of hours without committing errors! I prayed that none of my mistakes would be serious and that I wouldn't hurt anyone, including myself.

When you are tired, it is easy to make mental errors in judgment. Sometimes I confused patients and lab data. One patient can easily become entangled with the case next door because the chart racks are usually full.

It is also all too easy to stick yourself with a stray needle when you are in the middle of rushing to and fro doing procedures on numerous patients. Unfortunately, these "sharps" can carry the AIDS or hepatitis viruses. Fatigue is an occupational hazard in medicine, and it can be literally deadly for both the patient and for the doctor.

In a later chapter, you will learn that my prayers about mistakes were not always answered in the way that I would have liked. Because of one mistake that took a fraction of a second, my life has never been the same.

Sometimes I prayed to get home safely when my body just couldn't go any further. I was like a drunk stumbling home at:

Three A.M.

Three a.m. and it's just another night
Or is it daylight?
I'm disoriented, confused,
And my body feels abused.

Oh, I'm tired and worn,
And a little forlorn.
Lots of caffeine in my veins,
God! I had better switch lanes!

Rotations

Rotations are block periods of time spent studying specific areas of medicine. Some examples are internal medicine, surgery, their various subspecialties, and the emergency room. Most rotations require "night call," meaning that the doctor has to sleep in the hospital, answer emergency calls, take admissions, and see consults from other physicians. On some rotations, this meant sleeping in a bunk bed in the hospital every other night or sacking out wherever your body happened to land.

In the case of the intern, taking call would usually involve being awake for the most part of thirty-six hours. He or she would drive home, eat dinner, hopefully do something that could be compressed into minutes, and then finally collapse into bed at an early hour in order to report to the hospital at seven the next morning to prepare for rounds. Most of my own time away from the hospital was spent sleeping and eating. I sometimes just sat like a zombie in front of the television set. There was little quality time with friends or family. The worst thing of all was that there was precious little time for "**me.**"

All patients have charts that have to be buffed and prepared for presentation on rounds. These charts contain all the pertinent information about their cases: lab tests, progress notes, etc. During rounds, charts are polished instead of boots and buttons; it's essentially a medical version of a military inspection. The attending physician would come by and review his troops every day after morning report, making sure that everything was in its place.

In the case of some of Dr. DeBakey's surgical residents, having a social and marital life was virtually impossible. Some of his residents—those in what was called "the pit," or Fondren ICU—literally lived in the hospital for at least a month at a time. Their wives were allowed weekly conjugal visits, at which time the nurses were asked not to interrupt unless it was a dire emergency. Unfortunately, in this ICU, these visits didn't last long as emergencies occurred multiple times throughout the day. Needless to say, the conjugal visits themselves became emergencies!

There were few weekends off during my residency training. Several residents left Fondren ICU to find that their cars were either towed or stolen, that their marriages were disintegrating, or that their wives had plain run off. One unfortunate fellow named Sammy developed tuberculosis while working in "the pit." Several residents suffered from mental or physical exhaustion. Some dropped out and couldn't handle the pressure.

Fondren ICU has been a proving ground for surgical residents. When I was at Baylor, anecdotes were rampant about Dr. DeBakey's intolerance of mistakes. The housestaff learned early in their training that they had better be well prepared for his early morning rounds so that they could leave the best possible impression on their perfection-oriented teacher.

The doctors and nursing staff made sure that everything was in place. Sometimes the inspection would come as a surprise attack at 5 A.M. Dr. DeBakey had a reputation as an early riser. No one wanted to be the recipient of his anger or the source of his wrath. When he was angry, Dr. DeBakey could make Pearl Harbor look like a minor ambush. Nurses made sure that their patients were looking their best. Everyone who worked in Fondren I.C.U. was on his or her toes. You had to be; there was no choice!

The housestaff in the pit served their time and paid their dues in order to get the best possible recommendation for either the best fellowships (the next step beyond residency training) or for the best private-practice opportunities.

Complainers at Baylor did not fare well; therefore, publicly heard complaints were rare. The training experience was the ultimate test of endurance, like a triathlon. Most of us felt that it was a necessary evil, a "rite of passage" to the next level, something we had to endure. During my five years at Baylor, the stories of endurance were impressive, but so were the stories of depression, fatigue, and exhaustion.

It is important to understand that not only are interns and residents required to prove their medical skills to their instructors, but they also need to prove that they have physical and mental fortitude. Residency training has not only been a test of machismo, in which only the strong survive, but it has also been a weeding out process for the weak, or for those who just don't want it badly enough. My fellow interns and I were rushing the medical fraternity, and we had to prove that we wanted to join the club badly enough, no matter what happened to ourselves or to our loved ones in the process.

"E.R."—A Fast Track to "The Facts of Life"

Ben Taub's E.R. has been, and still is, one of the busiest emergency rooms in the country. It is literally inundated with sick people, many of them indigent and unable to afford medical care, which makes it a wonderful learning experience, a place for young doctors to practice medicine. It is also where the majority of trauma patients are taken in the downtown Houston area due to its reputation for being one of the busiest and best trauma centers in the country. Incredible pathology comes through its doors, and we saw things that would both help and haunt us for the rest of our lives.

The E.R. is also an example of an overwhelming experience by virtue of its sights and sounds. Walls are lined with patients on stretchers or sitting in chairs waiting to be seen after being "triaged." Being triaged means that the nursing staff weeds out the sicker patients from the ones that we could take our time with. The sicker patients were to be seen promptly (fast tracked) although this higher priority still didn't guarantee being seen by the doctor in less than four or five hours.

Patients were lined up out the door on Friday and Saturday nights, as if waiting to get a ticket to the movie theater. At first, I wondered if there was a magnet in the E.R., drawing people to its doors. I didn't realize how many sick people there actually were out there. How could we take care of all of them?

The E.R. was also my first experience with seeing man's inhumanity to his fellow man, as well as his transgressions. Gunshot and knife wounds were abundant; we often talked about the Friday and Saturday night "knife and gun clubs" and wondered whom its victims would be when we were on duty. Unfortunately, all too many of them were police officers and innocent bystanders.

It was also an experience in seeing victims of rape, abuse, and violence. Women would come in with tears in their eyes and be asked to spread their legs apart so that we could examine them and take semen specimens from their vaginas. Their physical and mental trauma became **my** trauma. The E.R. became a trauma center for the patients, their doctors, and their families.

I was forced to see the horror and waste of human life through the eyes of a parent's shock and grief at the death of her innocent child:

A Desperate Prayer

Where did she go?
She was playing outside a minute ago!
Where is she now? She's out of view.
I can't see her 'til they tell me to.

Helplessly waiting
Anticipating….
Doctors and nurses running everywhere
All of them wanting to help and care.

My God, blood is all that
my eyes Can see.
Don't let this be happening to me,
Or to her,
After all, she's just a little girl.

I can't stand this gruesome sight.
No, it won't be all right.
Her body, mangled and bare,
With blood-soaked hair.
Taken from me at the age of three,
It's not fair, it just cannot be!
To a bullet my child was prey,
Dear Lord, help us to find our way.

Busy surgical residents "cracked chests" and massaged the hearts of gunshot victims. They often couldn't wait for the opportunity to do what they had only read about in textbooks. Dr. Kenneth Mattox, the chief of staff and head of thoracic surgery, had a reputation for being one of the best surgeons and instructors in the country. He often came into the hospital on Saturday nights to help his residents learn the intricacies of opening chests and cross-clamping aortas.

"See one, do one, teach one" was sometimes the only way to learn in the E.R. The pace was fast and furious, and you had to jump right in, or you were left sitting on the bench.

Internal medicine interns and residents, such as myself, saw things that we would probably never again see for the rest of our lives. It was not unusual to diagnose cases of tuberculosis or gonorrhea at all hours of the day and night. We took care of at least ten overdose victims in a typical twelve-hour period, and we saw scores of others with diseases that we had only read about or had never even heard of.

It not only took fortitude to make it through the E.R., but it also took an ability to deal with all the repulsive sounds, sights, and smells that I had been exposed to and had hated in medical school. It required the development of a special "immunity" to seeing pain and suffering.

I found myself becoming hardened to the sights and sounds that inundated my daily existence in the E.R. Being surrounded by so much human waste and carnage can leave even a normal person mentally traumatized and shell-shocked. I found myself going from room to room just trying to keep up with a pace that seemed impossible. There was little time to talk and chat; sometimes there was little time to feel sorry for people. Faces and names became a blur, often becoming indistinguishable from one another. I functioned on autopilot; there was no choice.

Unfortunately, there was little time to show compassion, and I could feel it ebb, especially when the pace became frantic. There were even times when I wished that patients would just die or disappear so that I would just not have to deal with it all anymore. The drug overdoses wasted my time, and I actually got to enjoy pushing that big fat tube down their nostrils into their stomachs to pump out the pills that they had swallowed. "That will teach them," I sometimes felt. I knew that most of them would be back within a week and keep me busy again.

At the end of my shift, I was anxious to just escape into a world where no one complained and where there were peace and quiet. I often wanted to be by myself and listen to music or just escape into a dream world. I was literally drained of emotion and physically exhausted. This feeling was a harbinger of "things to come" in later years.

Young doctors saw people in all walks of life, ranging from "bag people" found on street corners to drug dealers, to policemen, and even to doctors and executives. The President of the United States would have been brought there if he had been shot while visiting Houston. The E.R. taught young doctors that illness and trauma didn't segregate between the social classes although most of the patients at Ben Taub were indigent, and many were even homeless. A lot of them were victims of society's ills.

People were sometimes literally found in dumpsters and were brought in by the E.M.S. (emergency medical service) so dirty and smelling so vile that we didn't want to touch them until we had gloved, masked, and thoroughly washed and deloused them. They usually were soaked in their own urine and smelling of the feces and vomit that had almost drowned them. On most of these occasions, I wanted to let the nurses and aides do the dirty work before I would even get close to the patient. Often they were too sick, and they couldn't wait to be cleaned and debugged first. The nurses were the doctor's first line of defense, and they were wonderful at both protecting us and at caring for our patients. We relied on them to warn us of trouble and to keep us out of harm's way!

As an E.R. doctor, you value your relationships with your coworkers, especially the nursing staff. Nurses could be your best friend or your worst enemy. You had best learn early that you don't "piss off" or upset E.R. nurses. These people are a special breed, and they thrive on what they are doing. You could learn a lot from them. On the other hand, interns who thought they knew everything or were arrogant could suddenly find themselves cleaning and delousing their own patients in all the confusion!

My respect grew daily for both the ambulance personnel (the Emergency Medical Technicians, E.M.T.'s), and for the nurses who fought the E.R. battles day in and day out throughout their careers. They saw more horror stories than I could ever dream about. Many of the patients were already stabilized by the time they came through the doors of the E.R. to see the triage nurses. We became a team that was built on mutual respect, or at least that was the way that it usually worked. Every so often, we had a doctor who wanted to be a showoff.

Tom was an intern who couldn't wait to show the veterans what he could do. He often brushed off the nurses' suggestions and one day found himself in a jam. Tom thought that he could do it all by himself and had something to prove.

One day, a heart-attack victim came into the E.R. and suddenly "coded," meaning that his heart stopped. Or at least that's what Tom thought. He misread the electrocardiogram (EKG) and shocked the patient while he was wide awake and with a totally normal heart rhythm. The nurses tried to tell him that he was making a mistake, but Tom just grabbed the paddles and applied a shock of four hundred joules to his patient's chest. The patient literally hit the ceiling. No one heard from Tom again for a long time.

It was a sad fact, but all of us in the E.R. knew that we couldn't cure society's ills or our patients' social problems. We often referred cases to social workers, who did their best, but most often we would clean them up, cure their physical problems, and then send them right back to where they came from. Alcoholics and drug addicts often went back out onto the street. We knew that a lot of them would come back. There were too many "repeat performers" in our American tragedy.

The E.R. developed a reputation for separating the men from the boys. For some of us, it was our first exposure to the sweetness of success and the agony of failure as doctors. It was where I learned that "Humpty Dumpty" is more than just a fictional character out of a fairy tale. Unfortunately, there are some people that I just couldn't put back together again, no matter how hard I tried. I almost fell apart myself.

Learning to Play a Dangerous Game

In the E.R., a doctor sometimes develops a reputation as either "**a rock**" or "**a sieve**," the latter being the doctor who allows the patients to pass through the pores of the E.R. to the hospital wards. They generally awaken the housestaff a lot throughout the night with admissions. When I was working the wards, I loved to work when "the rock" was in the E.R. because I felt safe and protected.

The number of sick people requiring hospitalization was simply staggering, and we prayed not to be overwhelmed with more people than we could physically care for. We were basically in a battlefield, and I was looking for the demilitarized zone where I could find an escape from the chaos and confusion. Times of peace and quiet in the E.R. were few and far between.

We all looked for ways to survive the battles and serve our time. A lot of residents liked the fast pace and intensity of the E.R. and eventually went into emergency medicine as their specialty. For me it was an experience that I will never forget, but I was ready to move on to other things.

The supply of beds was simply not enough to meet the demand of patients who waited in line for medical care and needed admission to the hospital. One way that "the rock" helped his fellow residents was by transferring the patient to other institutions, such as the VA Hospital, if he or she was an honorably discharged veteran, or to a private hospital if he or she had insurance. One of the first lessons that we learned during the E.R. rotation at Ben Taub was to look for insurance or veterans' cards in the patients' pockets and wallets. There was a feeling of relief if we could find any proof that the patient was eligible for transfer to someone else's care.

The process of transferring patients to another institution or to a different service is called "**turfing.**" Turfing has been an accepted practice because it lessens the housestaff's workload. It is not only tolerated but also rewarded with praises such as, "You did a great job turfing that patient to the V.A. Hospital!" Successful "turfers" have learned to play a game that is called "**dumping.**" Patients are literally dumped onto another medical service or hospital. There are a variety of methods to "turf," and most doctors have it down to a science. Knowing how to turf is as important to a Ben Taub resident as knowing how to start an I.V. You had to know how "to work" the system.

As with any other game, we became more experienced and better at it with practice. If my patient fell out of his bed and broke his leg during the hospital stay, then he was turfed to orthopedics. If he developed a surgical abdomen, then he was transferred to surgery. If we discovered he was a veteran, then he went to the V.A. Hospital, that is, as long as the hospital had a bed. My peers and I became very efficient with these transfers.

There were rules to play by, and none of us wanted to be called "dumpers." When I was an intern, the pressure to find a detour for patients was intense. The housestaff was usually swamped with numerous admissions during an ordinary night, and they were desperately looking for relief. There was also a lot of pressure to find peer approval from other doctors and being "a rock" was a way of gaining acceptance from your teammates.

One night I drove a patient from the Ben Taub E.R. to neighboring Hermann Hospital just to prove that I was a successful turfer and to gain acceptance from my comrades. My patient was in diabetic ketoacidosis and had gastrointestinal bleeding. He obviously needed to be admitted to the hospital. I put him in the front seat of my car, literally drove him around the block to the E.R. at Hermann Hospital, and presented him to its incredulous staff. The staff looked at me as if to say, "Are you in your right mind?" In retrospect I'm sure that my frame of mind was not "right."

This patient eventually received the care from others that he should have received from me. Although I had played the game successfully, this memory is one that I am not very proud of. I cringe when I even think about it. I had succumbed to peer pressure and had put a patient's life in possible jeopardy. I never repeated this mistake, but it still haunts me to this day.

The philosophy of proving one's toughness is an attitude that is ingrained in residents from day one. I felt that I couldn't show any sign of weakness. Proving my "toughness" became a code to live by, just as much as learning, eating, and sleeping. I wanted desperately to prove myself worthy of being a doctor, but more than anything else, I wanted to survive!

The residents tried to help the interns, but the unspoken philosophy of my training program was to "sink or swim." A person who couldn't handle the pressure either found a different career, a different specialty, or a different place to learn medicine. My indiscretion never was made known to any of my residents or attendings. Hopefully, somewhere along the line, I have discovered a way to put the patient first and a need for approval second. My ideals would no longer be compromised by my insecurities.

The Elegant Master

At Baylor I discovered what I nicknamed, somewhat irreverently, the "DeBakey Philosophy" of teaching medicine. It tests one's abilities to cope with adversity on a daily basis, be sleep deprived beyond endurance (and sometimes recognition), and still function to the satisfaction of one of the world's premier surgeons. Although this philosophy may sound archaic and even sadistic, it has produced some of the best doctors the world has ever seen.

My first experience with "DeBakey Rounds" is etched in my memory as vividly as if it happened yesterday. Dr. DeBakey entered the room in his blue scrubs, his surgical cap still pulled over his head, and his mask hanging below his chin. I had always wanted to touch Dr. DeBakey's velvety looking scrubs. They looked soft and gave him the appearance of royalty. They contrasted with a rather plain-looking face that was bespectacled and somewhat gaunt but made him look younger than his years. His eyes were dark and tired; they appeared to soak in everything around him. Nothing escaped his no-nonsense gaze.

The masterful surgeon had his back to us. The room was filled with cardiology fellows and attendings waiting to present their cases. He rarely looked at the people behind him. No one really wanted to make eye contact with Dr. DeBakey. His stern gaze could shake you to your feet. Everything had to be in order; the x-rays had to be in the right place, and the presenter had to be prepared to present a short, concise summary of the case. Dr. DeBakey was there to give advice, not to hear a lecture.

The time finally came for me to present my case. It took all of thirty seconds. Dr. DeBakey never looked up; he took notes about my patient and quickly went onto the next case. I breathed a sigh of relief and hoped that I would never have to come back.

Even as I was finishing my training, stories were rampant of verbal slashing that took place on "DeBakey Rounds" if everything wasn't just right. Whether they were fact or fiction doesn't matter. These rumors, along with his reputation, had the effect of intimidating almost everyone in his presence.

I admire Dr. DeBakey and consider him to be one of the hardest-working and gifted physicians that I have ever met. He routinely was at the hospital at all times of the day and night. He is the "Iron Man" or the "Lou Gehrig of Medicine." He expected the same dedication from those under his careful tutelage.

If Dr. DeBakey ever smiled or laughed, it was never in front of his housestaff and trainees. He was always the stern but aloof father figure for everyone around him. I admire the man greatly for his medical skills but have often wondered if he could not also have been kinder, more compassionate, a gentler father-figure to those whom he taught so much without relinquishing his quest for dedication. Most of us were not able to get close enough to Dr. DeBakey to see his warm side. Maybe he could not allow us to see anything else:

The Elegant Master

To the elegant master no one
can compare.
His gifts are so wondrous to
the human race
That the sick 'round the
world flock to his care,
To witness his healing, style, and grace.

Aging, bespectacled teacher,
dedicated and Aloof,
We are indebted to our father figure,
His talent and hard work we salute,
Thru his students, his greatness
will endure.

Craziness?

If one were to look up the definition of a "doctor-in-training," it might read something like: "An academic marathon runner, one who eats, sleeps, and breathes medicine and suffers from chronic fatigue and exhaustion; a person who borders on insanity and lives 'on the edge,' subjecting himself to things that most human beings would say 'no' to without much thought; an example of delayed gratification and obsessive-compulsive behavior; See also: 'workaholic.'"

Going through medical school is more than hard work. Taking call every other night in residency training is downright brutalizing. It can send the best of us over the edge. Some of my friends joked that taking call every other night actually caused us to miss half "the fun" and educational experience. Fair or unfair, it is part of the education of many of our doctors.

I both loved and hated the experience of becoming a doctor, and I know deep down in my heart that it was unhealthy for those who suffered through the ordeal along with me. Twenty years later, my feelings haven't changed. At times, it was a degrading experience, and I felt like an abused mule pulling the plow.

I don't agree that our current system is a necessary evil and short-term sacrifice that produces wonderful and healthy doctors. Tell that to a child who barely gets to see his father or mother for months at a time or to a spouse who is forced to deal with critical issues at home without his or her mate's help. I don't know if I could go through this craziness again or recommend it to my children.

However, a part of me also loved the challenges that were represented and special abilities that were created by my life of:

Craziness

Crazy hours, crazy days,
There's no end in sight.
I feel like a rat in a maze,
Who, desperately trying
With all his might,
Never reaches daylight.

Some doctors thrived on the experience that could be called "the making of a doctor." But none of us had a clue that we would be virtual prisoners of the system that was training us. Like so many other things in life, you can never quite understand an experience unless you actually "walk the walk."

The spouses of our housestaff had no idea what they were getting themselves into. For many of the spouses who had children, the experience was like single parenting. No one took the time to explain things to them up front and honestly. That is a problem that I hope to remedy with this book.

As for myself, nothing had really prepared me for the incredible adventure that I have undertaken for my life's work. Sometimes it has been a nightmare rather than the dream that was supposed to embrace me with happiness. My life has turned into a jumble of personal failures, miscalculations, and unfulfilled promises. Medicine is a very demanding mistress, and I underestimated the power of her not-so-gentle persuasion.

Publish or Perish

I finished my fellowship training in cardiology three years after finishing my residency training. I had gone to school and trained for a total of fourteen years after high school. After all that time, I felt that I had taken medicine's "best shot" and had survived the worst ordeal that I could ever envision for my young life. After all those years, I finally felt prepared to get out into the real world, spread my own wings, and fly above the tumult and chaos.

First, I had to leave the world of academic medicine. Not everyone was pleased with my decision. Interestingly, the Chief of Cardiology at Baylor College of Medicine chose to make an example of me to the entire group of fellows.

Just prior to my leaving the Baylor cardiology program, the chief of cardiology asked me a startling question during a seemingly routine meeting with the entire group of fellows. He asked me to explain my personal reasons for leaving academics to go into private practice. Unprepared for the question and shocked, I did my best to explain my feelings and my philosophy of how I wanted to help people deal with illness and cope with their problems.

His response shocked me even more. What followed was a lecture about the necessity of staying in academic medicine. His premise was that my reasons for leaving it were inadequate to justify my actions. At the time, I didn't argue with him; I played the game and wanted to preserve my future. I still relied on him to allow me to finish my training and get away from the clutches of such a stifling attitude.

It wasn't easy, but I bit my tongue and kept my mouth shut. However, the memory of his cynical and harsh rebuke left me with a hard-to-restrain contempt for his audacity to question a very personal and private decision that I had made and felt strongly about.

There is no question in my mind that he was trying "to round up the strays" by painting me as an example of the kind of doctor that he didn't want in his program. It was the old school of teaching at its best and worst. I represented the antithesis of his philosophy, a bug that he wanted to squash and an infection that he didn't want to have spread to others.

The idea of setting me apart as an example of "what not to do" came from his desire to prod other fellows into following the academic path that he had chosen for us. He was using me to set his priorities for the cardiology section, and since I was about to leave, I was expendable.

His actions were also an example of how doctors are indoctrinated. Intimidation is a common tactic because a fear of failure is part of the everyday life of a young doctor. Department chairmen know that they hold an awesome power over the lives of those that they teach. No resident wants to be "the black sheep" in the family. It's easy to succumb to such power. It would have meant academic suicide for any of us who dared to try to fight authority.

I am not writing out of bitterness or a desire for literary revenge. My mentors are characters in the play that has become my life. They have helped to mold me into what I have become, both as a person and as a professional. What has happened since then has been for the best. I made the best decision **for me**, which was to leave an arena where teaching is done through intimidation, hazing, and sleep deprivation to go into a totally different world, a world that would present an entirely new set of obstacles. I left behind those who wanted to stay in that environment so that I could find my own answers to life.

Thinking that I was leaving the worst behind me, I left my training and was excited about the new adventures that I was about to face. As I was soon to discover, my education was far from complete. My patients and my experiences were to become my greatest teachers.

Did We Fail Them?

Unfortunately, two more of my friends and classmates met premature deaths by taking their own lives. Kevin killed himself in the early morning hours with an overdose of potassium, a substance that can cause the heart to suddenly stop beating. We found him dead in the residents' workroom at the V.A. Hospital.

Jim shot himself after disappearing from his home in the wee hours of the morning. His wife frantically searched for him. We found him in the park with a bullet in his brain.

Both were outwardly normal functioning human beings but inwardly must have been going through an emotional "hell," unbeknownst to even their closest friends.

Twenty years later, I am still haunted by those terrible deaths. Something pushed them over the edge. I still wonder if we could have done anything to prevent the three people who committed suicide during my training from getting to the "point of no return."

Why didn't we realize that they were in such pain? Could we have been more sensitive to their plight? Were we too caught up in our own little worlds, caring only about our own survival? Could the long hours of sleep deprivation and pressure have caused these people to lose their ability to think rationally and to see no other way out? How did we get so blind to the needs of our friends? Was this all just a terrible coincidence? The answers never came, and I don't expect that they ever will.

I don't doubt that these individuals may have taken their own lives even if we had known that they were troubled souls. Underlying problems exist in a system that leaves too many people with a feeling that they have no other alternative but to end it all. The answers would logically seem to lie in creating a system of medical training that is based on compassion, not only for the patient but also for the doctor.

A scary statistic that emphasizes this problem is the fact that female physicians over twenty-five have a four times greater chance of committing suicide than women in the general population.[1]

Something is terribly wrong with a system that accepts this statistic of death as a fact of life. Women have their own terrible pressures to endure as doctors and have to prove themselves "tough" to survive in what had until recently been a male-oriented profession. Who really takes the time to understand their problems?

Instituting preventive measures is important, not just to decrease the suicide rate but also to produce healthier doctors who are less likely to also become drug addicts and angry, depressed individuals.

Changes have occurred in some medical training programs to make them more responsive to the needs of students, but I am skeptical that these changes have significantly reduced the intense pressure that is at the core of medical training. We are creating excellent doctors but omitting the one thing that the doctor needs to learn the most: how to compassionately care for his patients and for himself!

"Medical education in the United States today takes people who enter the system filled with humanism and idealism and ultimately forces them to surrender these ideals by the very process that turns them into technically competent and intellectually capable physicians."[2]

There needs to be a paradigm shift from the philosophy of "proving your endurance" to "showing your humanity." There should be a shift from "less sleep makes better doctors" to "sleep deprivation produces unhealthy human beings who place both themselves and their patients at risk of harm."

Since we are producing successful physicians who are among the best in the world, these changes will not come easily or without debate. My question to the leaders of medical education in this country is: "Can we afford to pay a cost that is so dear when the stakes are so high?"

Residency programs vary from place to place and from specialty to specialty. Medical training programs exist where student-doctors are more than just numbers, where learning is accomplished without severely intense pressure, and where there is a real interest taken in a person's humanity. Hopefully, in the future, programs will learn from their mistakes and allow an environment that is more conducive to healing the doctor, not just the patient.

The University of Texas family practice residency program in Conroe, Texas, teaches its students that it is important to have a strong work ethic but that your life's work should be fun at the same time. Other programs should model themselves after this example.

What Comes Next?

After reliving my experiences in this book, I am amazed that I survived the ordeal that is called medical training. It took great willpower and determination. The cost was exorbitant to my mind, body, and soul.

I left my training not only as a well-trained doctor but also as a naïve individual who had no compass or direction. Even though I had a new title, I didn't know "who" I was or where to find happiness.

Excelling in Delayed Gratification

I majored in English; I graduated with honors from medical school; I specialized in cardiology; but I excelled in delayed gratification. Eventually there certainly would have to be more time for both my family and for me. Wow, was I ever so wrong!

A constant refrain that echoed in my mind throughout the years has been:

"Just hang in there a few more years, and it's going to get easier, I just know it!"

I was the epitome of delayed gratification, and I was great at it! It was my "breakfast of champions!"

Part of what helped me survive the ordeal of my training was the belief that it was all going to get easier after I finished my residency and fellowship at Baylor College of Medicine. Certainly long nights and days of work had to yield to an easier schedule that I could control because I was going to be the boss! I realized soon after I entered private practice in a small town called Conroe, Texas, that I was about to be swallowed up by pressures of a totally different kind and that I was anything but my own boss!

Building a practice of any kind is hard work. It requires dedication and long hours of getting to know the people who will form your referral base. I hit the ground running, working twelve- to fourteen-hour days before coming home to take more calls at night.

There is also the business end of the practice that requires establishing contacts at banks with loan officers. There was no way that I could afford the huge outlay of cash that it would take to buy expensive medical equipment.

I was astonished to find that a treadmill could cost as much as twenty-five thousand dollars and that it costs thousands upon thousands of dollars to furnish an office. My ultrasound machine cost as much as my house!

Like most people starting a small business, I had to take loans to get my practice going, which was not a big problem as doctors were still considered by banks to be good risks during the early eighties.

I discovered that handling the business end of a medical practice was not an easy task. Taking care of patients does not leave a large amount of time to hire, fire, and make business decisions. I quickly began to delegate some of the responsibility so that my fourteen-hour days would not become sixteen-hour days. This later led to some catastrophically poor decisions and sometimes to just plain indecision.

I had headaches from the stress of trying to be a doctor and a businessman at the same time. During my training, no one ever taught us about dealing with disgruntled or dishonest employees, about paying back bank loans, and affording huge malpractice premiums. We were able to concentrate on taking care of sick people! Isn't that what being a doctor is all about? Now I was out in the real world of business where I had no shelter from a reality that faces millions of other Americans.

I quickly found out that the I.R.S. is more than just a short form and soon realized that life was easier when it was less complicated. I actually missed "the simple life" and hired someone to help with my pension plan and with I.R.S. regulations so that I would conform to all the rules and stay out of trouble with the government. The terrible thought of an audit did not seem inviting at all. Being a doctor was hard enough without that!

Learning the intricacies of health insurance and Medicare has been extremely complicated and frustrating. The rules of the game change almost daily, and it is almost impossible to keep up with all the things that you need to do to be compensated for your work.

It is entirely possible to work twenty-four hours a day and not get paid a cent because of incorrect coding and billing! And the managed-care industry makes it as difficult as possible to collect the money that is rightfully earned, often delaying payment to physicians for as long as the law permits, and sometimes even beyond. Our healthcare industry presents a challenge that has turned into a living nightmare.

Life was full of new revelations as I first went out on my own. Being a resident was a lot like college used to feel: a distant memory of times that seemed better and easier than they really were. Like childbirth, there has been amnesia for some of the harshness of a life that seemed to be fading in the distance. A new reality had set in. The problem was that I wasn't sure if I liked it after all those years of hard work. But my bed was made, and I had to sleep in it.

It didn't take long for me to realize that being my own boss seemed vastly overrated. I began to wonder if private practice was all that it was cracked up to be. Everyone else but me seemed to be in charge! I had worked long hours, striving to prepare myself for something for which I was totally unprepared!

Being your own boss is a two-edged sword. Independence is great, but I have hated the headaches and stresses that have come with the territory. When everything has gone smoothly, I have been tired but on top of the world. Unfortunately, that was not often in the very beginning.

Eventually the realization hit me that my "real boss" was a little box that was strapped to my belt and that followed me home each night: my beeper! This God-forsaken #%$# gadget had control over my life, often dictating when I ate, slept, went to the bathroom, and sometimes even when I had sex. My boss became a source of extreme frustration, and I tried on more than one occasion to drown it in the commode. It represented a way of life that I quickly came to resent. Its novelty wore off quickly.

Medical school and residency trained me to be a doctor, not a businessman. I have felt more comfortable with a stethoscope around my neck than with a calculator in my hand. It was only after I was thrust into the world of business that I began to realize how poorly I had been equipped to be an entrepreneur.

My training taught me how to be a doctor, not how to deal with Medicare, managed care, and the I.R.S. How could I be so naïve after over twenty years of schooling? How could I be so "book smart" and know nothing about surviving in the real world? I felt like a worm that had been put on the end of a fishhook, and there were lots of fish out there waiting to take a nibble!

I established a successful medical practice and gradually learned about the practical side of being a doctor. There was no choice. It was a gratifying feeling when I started to see the fruits of my labor. Unfortunately, my lack of understanding about business and life led to an awful lot of mistakes and miscalculations along the way. You are going to read about these in the coming chapters.

But first, it is important for you to understand what makes a doctor tick. It takes a lot more than fancy diplomas hanging on walls or even initials after a person's name. Let's take a few moments and see what it takes to both become and to be a doctor. What makes a person go through this ordeal that we call medical training, and what kind of person takes care of us afterwards?

Endnotes

1. Angres and Talbott, *Healing the Healer, The Addicted Physician* (Madison, Connecticutt: Psychosocial Press, 1998), pp.139–40.
2. Marion, *Learning to Play God* (A Fawcett Crest Book, 1991) p. 267.

CHAPTER 2

The Passion and the Pain

"And I say that life is indeed darkness save when there is urge, and all urge is blind save when there is knowledge. And all knowledge is vain save when there is work. And all work is empty save when there is love; and when you work with love you bind yourself to yourself, and to another, and to God. Work Is Love Made Visible"

K. Gibran, *The Prophet*

You've Got to Have Heart

Being a doctor is a labor of love. A person needs to have an innate passion that enables her to live through long sleepless nights, difficult training, and countless hours away from family and friends. It all enables her to deal with other people's problems when her brain is on overload—and still come back for more! If you're a doctor without "heart," it doesn't matter how bright you are or how hard you work.

I have often cursed at my beeper and have struggled valiantly against it in a fight to the finish. Realizing that I couldn't vanquish my foe, it dawned on me that I really wouldn't be happier doing something less meaningful or anything less challenging with my life. When you love what you do, it makes the hard times easier. When you are a doctor, those hard times come frequently, often daily. You either learn to "love it or leave it."

Being a doctor becomes a part of an individual's identity; it's in your blood. As I have grown older, however, being a doctor has become a smaller part of "who" I am. Something deep down inside of my soul needs whatever it is that being a doctor gives me, and I think that is the case for most doctors. But I also feel that I have a God-given gift to give others. But being a doctor has also exposed my weaknesses.

Good things usually don't come easy in life. That saying was never more apropos than when examining what a doctor goes through to hang his shingle and practice in the modern world. Medicine requires a commitment that at times borders on the insane. What possesses a person to be a doctor in the first place? Do you have to be possessed by demons or be called by God to wear a white coat?

I have often playfully asked my colleagues what they want to be "when they grow up." There are a lot of interesting answers because many of them are unhappy with managed care, or with "not having a life," and wonder whether the grass is greener on the other side.

Interestingly, I don't know anyone who has left medicine to go into another profession. There is a fire and a passion that accompanies "the birthing pains" of becoming and being a doctor. I admit that I often wonder whether a person can be addicted to the "high" of being a doctor and whether he or she could be a good doctor without the hardships and pain that come with the title.

In the Looking Glass

**"You may fool the whole world
down the pathway of life
And get pats on your back as you pass,
but your final reward will be heartaches
and tears if you've cheated the man in the glass."[1]**

A big part of our identity resides in the image that we see in our mirrors. It isn't easy to look at our reflections without trying to find rose-colored glasses and a little makeup to dull the harshness of the stark reality that sometimes stares us in the face.

To start with, it is important to know our roots. I was not given a gold stethoscope as a teething ring, and I, like every other normal child, hated going to the doctor's office. No one in my immediate family was even remotely involved in the medical field. I was the first and quite possibly may be the last.

My parents were hard workers who instilled the same work ethic in both my sister and me. I was born into a Jewish family, and I am proud to be a second-generation American. Many of my ancestors sacrificed everything they had, fleeing persecution from communism and escaping from Hitler's concentration camps.

My parents and grandparents saw in America a land of opportunity, and they quickly decided that these opportunities were best obtained by getting an education. Becoming **"my**

son, the doctor" was the fulfillment of not only an American dream but also an immigrant's dream.

My sister's successes in school gave me, as the younger brother, a little more to prove and a little more impetus to strive even harder. She eventually became an attorney, and it is probably no coincidence that I have had a competitive relationship with attorneys ever since, although this has sometimes been painful and not always to my liking.

I attended Rutgers College in New Jersey, following in my dad's and my sister's footsteps. I did well and graduated with honors in English and was a Phi Beta Kappa scholar. The tradition of educational excellence continued. But wait, it's not that easy to follow in the path of excellence and to be what other people want you to be.

It takes talents and abilities that are far more important than just intelligence to be a good doctor. Let's look beneath the surface and find out just which elements can help a doctor be a hero and which ones can make him dangerous and even a menace to his patients.

I am going to take a few moments and dissect a doctor. You're not squeamish, are you?

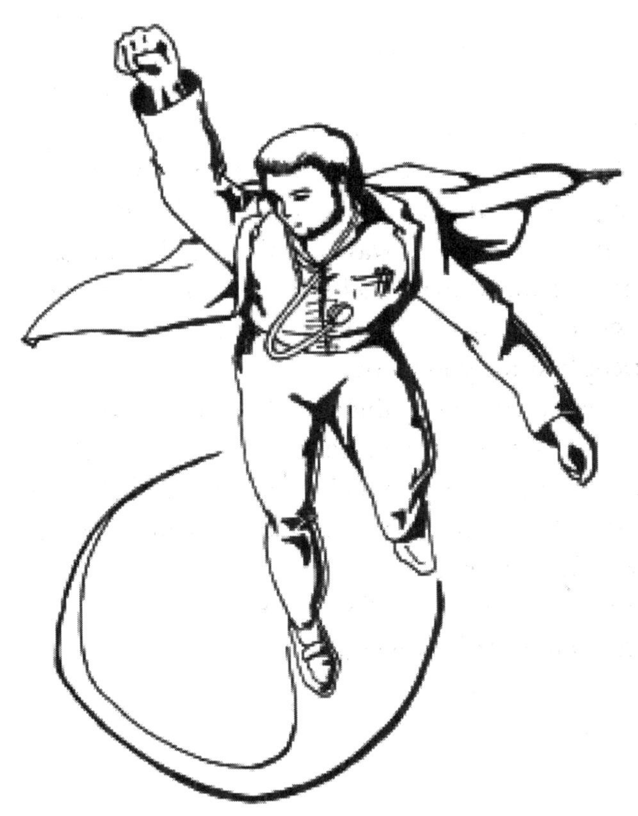

SAINT OR SUPERHERO?

"Being Able to Leap Tall Buildings in a Single Bound..."

Being Superman, or at least a superhero, helps when you're a doctor. Being able to be in more than one place at one time is an asset, and I have often thought of cloning myself. Super abilities are expected of doctors, and they often have a hard time living up to the advance billing and expectations.

Instead of changing my clothes in a phone booth, I have chosen more conventional accommodations, such as a restaurant or movie theatre restroom. I often imagine that I am Clark Kent being called to save someone in distress, and like mild-mannered Clark, I have had to literally change my appearance and demeanor in a hurry and rush off to the next rescue. There are times when it seems like the whole world needs my help! I'm Superman in scrubs and a white coat: Superdoc!

Doctors need to be able to switch gears in a split second. They need to be able to leave a dream fantasy in the middle of the night or a party with friends and rush to the hospital within a matter of moments. When a person is half asleep, it helps to be able to leap tall buildings in a single bound (or in my younger years, to sober up quickly). I never imagined that Superman had to leave parties and dates behind to save the world.

But alas, even Superman has his kryptonite. We'll discuss doctors' hidden weak spots later.

The Competitive Fire of Michael Jordan

A need to compete and win is not only a huge advantage, but it is also a necessary ingredient in the making of a doctor. The competition starts in high school and never stops! It is there every step of the way because the number of people who want to be doctors simply is far greater than the number who can be accepted into medical school. It's simple arithmetic.

Along the way, someone is always there to remind you that you may not make it. An inner voice is often whispering, "You had better try harder! You can't fail!" There are people who tell you that the odds are stacked against you and that the competition is fierce.

A competitive fire is necessary to get through the long hours of training and the intense emotional stresses of academics and daily living. It really doesn't get easier as you go to the next hurdle. The hurdles only seem to get higher and closer together!

I have competed almost every day of my life, but the competition has changed to a different playing field. The competition is now against disease, death, and managed care. I have been forced to adopt more competitive strategies that will allow me to survive in the managed-care marketplace that has become modern medicine. Stop and think about how much of life is based on the need to compete in a variety of forms.

Competition is internal for us obsessive-compulsive perfectionists. There is a need not only to succeed but also to succeed "perfectly." Over the years, my desire for perfection has yielded to a healthier and more peaceful philosophy: "Perfect is the enemy of good." But it took time and experience to get to that point, and also failure.

Over the years, I have come to understand that a lot of people need successful competition in order to feel good about themselves. Becoming a doctor was just what the doctor ordered for my ego. The same ego, however, caused me to take my failures seriously and to heart.

I hated "losing" to anything and anybody. I had to learn that "losing" is a part of life and that losing is often essential in order to understand and appreciate winning. This was a difficult and painful lesson to learn. It required admitting that I was human and that I couldn't change everything.

Competition not only makes you better at what you do but also stronger. However, too much emphasis is placed on competition in our society. The focus should be not so much on individual achievement but on creating doctors who are mentally and physically capable of treating others' problems without having an overabundance of their own.

We need to keep the competition healthy by focusing on competing against disease rather than on competing against each other.

A Quest for Perfection (*Mission Impossible*)

Let me restate a fact that has become obvious to me over the years: Doctors tend to be perfectionists and to be very compulsive about what they do. There is little margin for error because the stakes are so high. Incredibly strong self-discipline is essential and demanded by teachers, by peers, and by the profession itself.

There are a number of professions that can literally occupy a person's waking life and be all consuming and even suffocating. Medicine, as a profession, weeds out people who are not "Type A" personalities. The "trial by fire" of medical education won't allow people to be too laid back.

Let's face it! Don't you want your doctor to be a perfectionist? Would you still go to him even if he went out and played golf three days a week, didn't bother to show up to see his patients, or settled for mediocre results from his treatment?

Would you want your facelift or coronary bypass to be anything less than perfect? Would you go to a doctor if you knew that he or she had a reputation for being less than thorough? The answers to these questions are obvious and quite emphatic for most of us.

Medicine rewards obsessive-compulsive behavior because it demands long hours of study, hard work, and a preoccupation with details, rules, organization, and schedules. There is no way that I could have survived my training or my medical practice without being a compulsive workaholic. I had to be organized, meticulous, and disciplined about the way that I studied and performed my duties.

Unfortunately, many doctors get so caught up with the details of information gathering that they "lose sight of the forest for the trees." They get absorbed and distracted by minutia. People become sets of biological cells and a list of differential diagnoses rather than human beings with needs and feelings.

Medicine requires a devotion to work like few other professions. It is a jealous mistress who seeks all of the attention and energy of those who know her. It is hard to say "**No**" to her seductive powers.

By its very nature, medicine allows its students to be self-destructive. It is easy to hide behind the white coat, hide behind the long compulsive hours, and become numb to solving one's own problems. Society rewards doctors who work long hours and calls them "devoted." Everyone wants to go to a devoted and dedicated doctor. But that devotion extracts a price that has to eventually be paid.

Doctors can literally become slaves to their medical careers. They want to become the "best that they can be." Hard work and devotion, to the exclusion of other important things in life, are the pathways to success. "Working to live" is replaced by "living to work" as a way of life. It is easy for priorities to become confused and shifted.

Because of my extreme dedication to work, medicine allowed me to ignore important personal issues that I will talk about in later chapters. I was able to hide a variety of problems behind the white coat, including low self-esteem, difficulty with long-term relationships, and a lack of strong spiritual beliefs.

Eventually these problems caught up with me, and I could no longer hide behind the long hours and the hard work that ironically had become a refuge. Although I didn't realize it, the white coat had become my hiding place and refuge.

While I patted myself on the back, thinking that I was a noble, self-sacrificing human being, I was in reality practicing another art that I had perfected: self-deception. It took me almost twenty years to see beneath the camouflage that had been created by the initials that came after my name.

Medicine entices people who are compulsive by nature and trains them to perfect that talent by being compulsive about their profession. It lures people with a powerful aphrodisiac that feeds their needs and that sometimes hides their weaknesses and inner pain from the view of others, including themselves.

We need not to let go of our quest for perfection but rather to realize that we are human beings capable of making errors and then forgive ourselves for our frailties and mistakes. Anything else is *Mission Impossible* and can only lead towards unhappiness and sleepless nights.

I pride myself on being very meticulous about the standard of care that I give my patients and couldn't live with myself at the end of the day if I gave them anything less than my best. But I have tried to remember that I am far from indispensable and hope that I have become a little more of a Type B than a Type A personality. I no longer want to be imprisoned in my own mind by trying too hard to be something that I was never intended to be: perfect.

As a doctor, I have also realized that "work begets more work." The harder I work, and the longer my hours, the more work I create! It seems to multiply. What more would a compulsive perfectionist need to fulfill his dreams?

Have you ever seen a leopard change his spots? It isn't easy for any of us. We cause our own pain while trying to be like the artist who wants perfection in his masterpiece. Instead we create our own "living hell" by demanding too much from ourselves, and sometimes from others.

The Compassion of Mother Teresa

I once had a professor in medical school tell me that to be a good doctor you have to intuitively "like people." Can you imagine making your living taking care of people if you hated being around them? It definitely would be a miserable existence.

Let's face it! Most patients want their doctors to be like good parents: caring, comforting, and nurturing. Sometimes I think that my patients look upon me as a father figure! Why else would they confide in me things that most people would only tell their priest, rabbi, minister, or parent?

Obviously, the end result can be a huge disappointment. It's hard to be like Mother Teresa. If it were easy, then we would all be saints. Sometimes compassion is a hard thing to come by. I found that out when I was a houseofficer, when I would have traded my soul for a good night's sleep.

Compassion is a natural result of liking people and caring about them:

"Compassion is a feeling deep within ourselves—a 'quivering of the heart'—and it is also a way of acting—being affected by the suffering of others and moving on their behalf."[2]

Compassion, as an emotion, leads to action.

"It reinforces charity, empathy, and sympathy."[3]

This is an important catalyst for a physician and a big source of the fire and zeal that makes what he does a labor of love.

Frequently there are days when doctors are "burned out" from listening to the problems of others and want nothing more than peace and quiet. The last thing that they want is to see another human soul. This syndrome has a name and is called "burnout." It is a doctor's worst enemy.

There are ways to strengthen a person's ability to show compassion. Some of these involve mental and physical exercises, reading, and meditation. To be compassionate to others, a doctor (or anyone else for that matter) needs to be compassionate with himself first!

My feelings towards others are part of who I am, and there are times that I'm not successful at suppressing them. It's hard to be compassionate with someone who wakes you up in the middle of the night, and at times I have said to myself, "That person had better be dying, or he is on my shit list!" I'm human, like everyone else, and I often resent anyone who wakes me out of a sound sleep.

TLC in the proper doses is the best medicine that doctors can give, both to themselves and to their patients. It can also hide a host of sins and faults.

Then there are doctors called pathologists, who seem to prefer being around people who can't tell them about their troubles, except posthumously. I guess dead people can't wake them up at night!

The Courage and Heart of Lance Armstrong

Have you ever watched the "Tour de France?" Chances are that if you are an average American, you didn't watch it before Lance Armstrong came along. This man overcame cancer to win one of the world's most grueling and demanding races.

The "Tour de France" is a lot like life. You have to ride on all kinds of surfaces. There are a lot of ups and downs and curves in the road. You have to be more than good to win. It takes courage and a strong desire just to make it to the finish line. You can lose one leg of the journey one day and still come back and win the overall event. Being able to overcome adversity and bounce back is a necessity in life. That is especially true for doctors.

We all have our marathons to run. We choose some, and some choose us, whether we like it or not. The patient with cancer undergoing chemotherapy is running his marathon every day that he goes through the weakness, hair loss, and vomiting that accompanies his treatments. The patient who has just undergone bypass surgery is running his own marathon as he recovers and basically starts to live life over again.

Some marathons are longer and harder than others, but how we run them defines us as human beings and defines our characters. Both being and becoming a doctor is a marathon, one that seems endless. I was tempted to quit on more than one occasion and yell as loud as I could, "Stop the world, I want to get off!"

Doctors usually choose to run their marathon. It's just that they sometimes don't know how long the race is until they have left the starting block. Many don't realize that they picked a lifelong "Tour de France" until they have gone so far that there is no turning back.

The goal is to make it to the finish line happy, in one piece, and with your sanity intact. Several elements are crucial in allowing us all to face up to life's challenges; whether we are doctors or not is not important. First:

- We have to have courage and faith in ourselves. We need to believe in ourselves in order to run the race in the first place.
- Stamina, commitment, and perseverance are essential in helping us get to the finish line when we feel that we are about to give up.
- We have to get rid of our "excess baggage" and lighten our loads. We can't run if we are carrying the weight of

the world on our shoulders. If something is dragging us down, then we need to deal with it and free ourselves from the albatross around our necks.

- A cardinal rule of racing is "never to look behind you." We have to keep our eyes on the goal or we lose our momentum. That means learning from our mistakes and then going forward. That has been one of the hardest lessons for me to learn as a doctor. It is difficult to forget a mistake when it affects a human life. I have had to evaluate my mistakes then put them in their place and not carry them with me as excess baggage. I'll talk more about this subject later.
- We all need to understand that we are not running the race by ourselves. We need to have family and friends rooting us on along the path. We also need faith that someone is with us every step of the way. It's especially important to have spiritual faith when other human beings fail us.

I want to be able to say, when all is said and done, that I ran the best race that I could run and that I ran a race that I could be proud of. My motives for running the race will really not be all that important when I reach the finish line as long as I feel good about how I got there.

For doctors, every day can be a mini-marathon. They have to put it all on the line with every patient. One of the purposes of this book is to help doctors overcome the obstacles in their paths and get to the finish line in one piece.

The "True Grit" of John Wayne

Just a few words about grit and determination: These attributes have come in handy when I was about to give up and say, "Forget it!" Deep down I have always wanted to be a hero like John Wayne, coming over the hill with the cavalry to save the day!

There is nothing more satisfying than finishing a job successfully after failing initially, when the odds seem stacked against you. Opening up a badly blocked artery is one of the greatest feelings that I have ever experienced, and it is made all the more wonderful by the difficulties and obstacles that were overcome in the attempts. Making a difficult diagnosis is a reward that is even sweeter because someone's life will be better off because of hard work and stick-to-itiveness.

Some of my ancestors' stubbornness and determination have certainly found their way into my genetic makeup. I don't give up easily; would you want your doctor to give up after the first, second, or even third try at fixing your heart?

Doctors can't afford to lose too often; they are programmed to succeed early in medical training. Being a doctor takes determination, perseverance, and a personality that says, "It ain't over till the fat lady sings."

"The Duke" never quit. He had tenacity, even when he got a few bad reviews. It takes perseverance and determination to bounce back from adversity when things look the bleakest. On a lonely Saturday night when your friends are out partying and you are taking care of an E.R. full of patients, it's easy to wonder what the heck you're doing with your life.

The Confidence of Muhammed Ali

Would you want to go to a doctor who doesn't look at least outwardly confident about what he is doing? I'm not talking smug here. I think most of us would have difficulty entrusting our lives to someone who appeared to lack strength and conviction or seemed uncertain and insecure about his or her abilities.

It is important for a doctor to be self-confident in order to build his or her patient's confidence. But this outward show could be misleading and sometimes mistaken for arrogance.

There is a fine line for a doctor to walk, inspiring faith and confidence without an overabundance of pride or boastfulness.

I'm not suggesting that doctors necessarily have to talk like Muhammad Ali, but it is better than sounding like they don't believe in themselves. Besides, a little flashiness doesn't hurt!

Life has taught me not to get too cocky about my successes. Before I know it, I am brought back down to reality. I may get a wonderful "high" from the beautiful results of an angioplasty only to have everything go wrong the next time around doing the same procedure. Practicing medicine can be a very humbling experience. The saying, "Practice makes perfect" applies as much, if not more, to doctors as it does to others. The more I perform a particular procedure, the more confidence I develop in my capabilities and, simply put, the better I get.

Doctors subconsciously pass on their feelings of confidence to their patients in their mannerisms and body language. Patients pick up on these subtleties. They read a lot into what isn't spoken

It's very hard to fake confidence, although I did just exactly that when I was an inexperienced and insecure young doctor. In my earlier years of practice, I became a good actor because it was important to have my patients believe in me. It was also because I didn't want them to see the insecurities that I felt beneath the surface.

My initial experiences with medicine were indeed very humbling, and it is a wonder that I continued to pursue a medical career in spite of them. I worked my way through college as an O.R. (Operating Room) technician.

Learning how to hand surgeons the correct instruments that they need sometimes requires being a mind reader, especially when you don't understand what they are doing in the first place. It was an experience that I appreciated because it taught me not only about how hospitals worked but also a lot about some of the people who work in them.

My early memories of doctors were not very impressive, and the nurses looked at us as subhuman or like viruses, reminiscent of when I was an intern. Instruments were flung at me from a few of the angry surgeons. I left the job thinking that doctors and nurses were an egotistical and arrogant lot without any tolerance for mistakes or another's feelings (or at least mine). I left wondering why I had become a pre-med and asking myself whether this was really the world that I wanted to live in.

Fortunately, the passage of time has given me a different perspective on things. This early lesson taught me never to forget to treat those around me with respect, especially the people who hand me sharp instruments in the operating room!

Good doctors who know their limitations don't need to be arrogant or smug! Patients appreciate when I admit that I don't know everything and when I don't try to "con" them. They understand that I have the confidence without the unbearable ego to do the right thing when it comes to looking out for their best interests. Doctors need to mix the right blend of confidence with the understanding of the word "humility."

It helps to get in front of a mirror and practice saying, "I float like a butterfly and sting like a bee!" A little bit cocky may not be that bad after all.

But people can usually tell the pretenders from the contenders.

The Ability to Communicate Like Dale Carnegie

Without this, you might as well forget the rest! It is so important that I am going to discuss it in several sections of this book.

Communication is the ability to convey ideas effectively to another person. My father taught the Dale Carnegie course in public speaking. I originally scoffed at the idea that people wanted to take the time to learn how to speak. I later added it to the list of courses that I wish I had taken in school that would have helped my career and with life in general.

Dale Carnegie's book, *How to Win Friends and Influence People,* should be on every doctor's bookshelf. Being a good communicator is part of the art of being a good doctor, and it can be mastered with practice.

In order to communicate effectively with others, you first have to be comfortable with yourself. The self-confidence developed by effective speaking can be a great asset to a doctor. But first, it is necessary to understand the importance of communication in what we do as doctors. "It's not only what we say but how we say it" that is crucial.

How we write is also important. "The mark of a good doctor is usually illegible," according to John Kelly. He really wasn't kidding!

Most doctors, including myself, take and must pass a course in "How to Write Illegibly 101." I have spent time trying to analyze whether this trait is a genetic and/or learned tendency, and I have concluded that it is a combination of both.

Doctors are almost universally poor writers. Why? Maybe it adds to our mystique, or we are in a hurry, or maybe we just don't want to be understood at times. In my own case, my training as an English major didn't save me from my fate. I have often asked myself:

Why Can't I Write?

I am a doctor, I know
I am bright.
But words that sound so true,
Hide from sight,
And won't be read
In black or blue.

I can speak, hear, and read,
I hold words very dear too.
So why can't I write
So that others can read?
What a pity my words hide
From view!

The truth is that sloppy writing is just another example of poor communication. It is dangerous for both the doctor and his patients. Poor penmanship also gives attorneys more fodder for lawsuits and causes prescription errors.

Then there are doctors who actually write books even if they can't write legibly.

A Need to Go "Where No Man Has Gone Before"

Like Captain Kirk and Spock, doctors have a need for spirited adventure into new and uncharted territories. Every day is a day of new revelations and exploration. New knowledge surfaces, and better techniques to fight disease are found almost daily. Medicine is truly a voyage into the future of mankind.

Doctors have a need for discovery. The unknown beckons us with its call. We never know enough and are always learning. Every moment is a look into the crystal ball, and the wonders of the universe never cease to amaze me. Each day is different and offers new glimpses into what lies ahead of us. Brave new worlds and civilizations await us, and doctors are at the forefront of these adventures.

The Patience of "Job"

Patience and understanding are essential for a doctor. It isn't easy to listen to people's complaints day in and day out, especially when you have a few gripes of your own. I literally hear everything, from detailed recollections of bowel movements to problems with marriage, sex, and children. And I am a cardiologist, not a psychiatrist! People usually just want an ear to listen. They don't care about your title or your specialty.

The reality is that doctors need to listen to their patients in order to be effective. Conversely, in order to listen, they must be patient. Doctors are often guilty of not listening and have a reputation for being intolerant and impatient. We are looked at as being too busy for our own good. That is how society has judged us, and quite frankly, they are right about this one. But please read the rest of this book before you hand down the final verdict.

Many patients are obsessed with their problems. They worry about them day and night and often expect me to do the same. The result is that I lose sleep when they call, and I get grouchy. A vicious cycle starts; I stop listening and my brain turns off so that I can get some rest.

A person's patience is truly tested when patients call in the middle of the night about things that could have obviously waited until the next morning. Sometimes they are reacting out of fear and anxiety, but there are people who just insist on calling at their own convenience, perhaps to avoid the cost of an office visit. People often call at night because they know that they can talk to the doctor personally instead of to his or her staff. When this happens, which is often, I feel "taken advantage of."

Sometimes I receive calls from people whom I don't even know and who don't know me. They usually want free medical advice for themselves or for a friend. A lot of people want me to diagnose their problems over the phone, which is dangerous for them and a liability for me. It's also just plain impossible in a lot of situations to know what's happening without seeing a person in the flesh.

The majority of my calls and visits are from legitimately worried patients. I receive these twenty-four hours a day, seven days a week. Sometimes, I am half asleep when I talk to them and can't remember what I told them when I awaken the next morning. I try to be sympathetic, but it is hard when you are tired and want sympathy yourself. You just do the best you can and hope that it's good enough.

We need ***the patience of "Job"*** to help us when we reach the threshold of our endurance and when we just can't bear to hear one more complaint. Sometimes doctors must listen beyond what their endurance can tolerate.

Professionalism: A Brief Experiment with Noncomformity

As a patient, I want to go to a doctor who inspires confidence by the way he acts and dresses. I have seen a few doctors dress like someone out of *Gentleman's Quarterly*, and many of my colleagues look like someone out of a Levi Jeans advertisement, which is much more common in Texas.

When I was a medical student, I was taught to wear a shirt and tie under my white coat every day that I rounded on my patients in the hospital. It was deemed the "professional" appearance, an honored ritual, and part of the rite of passage to becoming a full-fledged doctor.

When I did a sub-internship at Grady Memorial Hospital, in Atlanta, I was surprised to see that residents in the south wore tee shirts and jeans. They thought I was just a hotshot kid from Philadelphia who was snobbishly showing off that he was a doctor-to-be. It was as if I was from a totally different culture, and I was!

Whether you wear jeans or dress like someone out of *G.Q.* is none of my business, and is not the issue. I am not advocating a particular dress code for doctors, but I have had experience with patients' expectations.

How a doctor dresses should depend on the situation and location. No one really cares how you look at 3 A.M. when you run into the emergency room to take care of her heart attack. In times of crisis, people just want a good doctor who knows what he or she is doing. Everything else takes a back seat.

I once tried an experiment by wearing an earring and a ponytail while I was in my early years of private practice. I will leave it up to you to decide whether this was part of a mid-life crisis, a last vestige of early rebellion, or a combination of both. I asserted my independence but at some cost. Some of my patients switched to other cardiologists in the area because they didn't want to go to a doctor who wore an earring.

Conroe is somewhat of a conservative little town in southeast Texas, where rednecks are not uncommon, and there is a town next door called "Cut and Shoot." By the way, the earring and ponytail didn't last long; I guess I thought I was in California! I learned that it is important to go with the flow. There were other ways to express myself.

The moral of the story is that doctors should dress in a way that inspires confidence in their patients and that they should look professional. Exactly what is "professional" is dictated by patients' expectations and by circumstances. People like to have a physician whose demeanor and appearance are positive influences in the healing process. They need to feel comfortable enough with a person to entrust him or her with their lives and innermost secrets. A doctor's ability to "win friends and influence people" by the way he or she looks and speaks is very important to his or her success.

I have learned the importance of people's perceptions. We can't ignore them just because we are doctors; if anything we need to be even more sensitive to people's feelings. We can't live in our own little worlds, no matter how tempting it is. How we present ourselves to others often dictates how effective we are at achieving our goals. I learned that the hard way. My brief experiment was a failure.

The Intelligence of Albert Einstein

Actually intelligence is the least important of all the things that are required to be a good doctor. Doctors don't necessarily have a higher I.Q. than the average voter; they just work harder than the average person to succeed. Let me emphasize two points: one is that being smart is vastly overrated, and the second is that it is not as necessary as other characteristics that I look for in my own family physician and in my colleagues.

Don't get me wrong. It is very important for a doctor to be smart, and it's an admirable trait. But a person can be intelligent and not be up on the latest techniques or, for that matter, care about their patients' feelings or welfare.

In the race between the tortoise and the cocky hare, I will take the slow and sure tortoise any day because I know he will get the job done and eventually finish the race. It is important to remember that "genius is 99 percent perspiration."

Having "smarts" may be just enough to get you "outsmarted." It doesn't make up for a losing personality or a poor bedside manner either. Patients want their doctors primarily to be affable, available, and compassionate. Many of them rank intelligence lower on the priority list. The simple truth is that people often don't care how much you know if you are someone they can talk to.

A Doctor's Kryptonite

No, I'm not talking about lawyers; they have their own special place in this book. Doctors have their own kryptonite; the pressures of the outside world often sap their strength and can even demoralize them, exposing their weaknesses. Let's examine the personality traits that can be self-destructive for doctors and which can transform them from superheroes into super villains in a hurry.

An Inability to Cope with Anger and Frustration

Frustration is what happens when reality collides with expectations. By that definition, doctors are inherently frustrated individuals. The reality of being a doctor is quite different than most people think it is.

If you are thinking about becoming a doctor, don't go into medicine expecting to make millions, to retire at a young age, to have an easy marriage, to have people automatically love and respect you because of your title, or that helping people is always rewarding and comes naturally. On the contrary, helping people is darn hard at times, and it takes a lot of delayed gratification and patience to be able to help your fellow human beings as a doctor.

My expectations are still colliding with the realities of my profession. I knew that medicine would be a demanding career, but I had no way of knowing that it would virtually control my life.

Twenty years ago, there was no way of knowing that managed care would give doctors gray hair or that medicine would have the distinction of being the oldest and most regulated non-governmental profession in our society…that is, of course, other than prostitution. That does make you pause to think, doesn't it?

Despite the fact that no one forced me to become a doctor, I am angry that my life has become so regimented and at times one-dimensional. There are times that I have been so angry that I have even taken it out on the wrong people, namely my kids and family. And then I get angry at myself for "losing it."

I found the answers to my frustrations and anger in the awareness of my career's hidden treasures:

Hidden Treasures

Our lives are full of hidden treasures,
Threads of beauty, veins of gold,
Offering feelings that are beyond measure,
That to one's heart can never grow old.

Seeing a baby cry for the first time,
Opening an artery, helping one mend,
Saving another's life,
And at the same time, mine,
This feeling of heaven, never let it end.

Treasures and frustrations,
How can one deal with such
Tears and elation?
That on earth a soul can barely touch?

The Control Freak

Some doctors just won't listen to another point of view. They feel threatened by the thought of being contradicted. This characteristic stems partly from the competitiveness and compulsiveness that is nurtured during medical training as doctors strive to emulate the attributes of their teachers, both good and bad. They are taught that doctors are supposed to be "in control of things." Patients generally want doctors who take charge. Society teaches us that our doctors are leaders who should be questioned but looked to for guidance.

Physicians who want to exert their dominance by controlling others generally don't do well with suggestions from their patients about alternatives. It's "my way or the highway," and there is little exploration of choices and viewpoints.

They usually feel threatened by requests for second opinions, and their patient's well-being suffers as a result. When they are asked to give second opinions, they are often very negative about the care of other doctors. Their insecurity lines the pathway to the courthouse both for themselves and for others.

I would love to say that I was never like this. When I left my training, I wasn't sure if I could handle the daily stress of making life and death decisions. The only way for me to cope with the pressure was to "take control." It was a defense mechanism that had its assets and drawbacks, but it defended me from my hidden insecurities and low self-esteem.

People with low self-esteem generally need to be in control of situations in order to function. Doctors are no different; insecurity manifests itself in the doctor who just can't listen to another viewpoint. This can be a very dangerous doctor.

Time has a way of teaching us humility and alternatives. Taking charge of the situation is good at the right place and time. But sometimes we have to learn when to back off and let others voice their opinions, or even do it their own way.

False Gods and Spiritual Isolation

During my youth, I didn't see a need for God in my life, and I didn't understand the importance of God to others. Like many "men of science," I felt that religion was the antithesis of the slide rule and the test tube. I didn't adhere closely to any particular religious traditions except when I was with my family. I attended and graduated from Hebrew School, and I was well versed in Judaism.

Although I was brought up around some beautiful traditions, I never felt a need to conform to the religious customs that were important to my family. My parents tried in vain to teach me the importance of having a strong belief in God, but I was too busy studying and rebelling against authority to understand their reasons.

I prayed instead to false gods: the gods of science. Many of my close friends did the same. I didn't need anybody else's help. After all, everything that was taught in my science and philosophy classes could get me through the problems of life. God became extraneous.

It took me years to discover just how wrong I was. I learned that it doesn't matter if a person's beliefs are of a Jewish, Christian, Buddhist, Hindu, or Moslem origin. For that matter, these beliefs could be alien and from outer space; the important point is that they exist and are there for people in their times of need.

Patients need their doctor's support from a spiritual standpoint. Physicians need to open the door to that option because many patients rely on religion, such as the chronically ill. Instead of ignoring the question, doctors need to address it tactfully with a question such as, "What gets you through the tough times in your life?" If spirituality or religion is the answer, then doctors can also ask, "What can I do to support or address spiritual or religious issues in your life"?[4]

Doctors sometimes just feel uncomfortable with the subject of spirituality and are afraid to discuss it with their patients. We need to understand that it is an important part of the healing process.

Solitary Confinement

One of the hazards of working long hours is that it cuts you off from friends and loved ones. At times, I have felt like I am in solitary confinement. Medicine makes it possible to live in your "own little world," cut off from others who are important in your life, and allows you to stay isolated from reality. As a result, doctors are subject to delayed development in other areas. I have labeled this phenomenon "social retardation."

I don't think that social retardation is at all uncommon, and it happens to the best of doctors. Some people might say that doctors have our heads so high up in the clouds that we have never learned how to relate to people on the ground. As a result, doctors sometimes learn things later in life than the people around them.

Being socially isolated doesn't create a bad doctor unless it leads to depression, substance abuse, anti-social behavior, or addiction. Social isolation may cause difficulty with personal and professional relationships.

I spent the most part of twenty-five years of my life in intense study and hard work preparing me for what was ultimately my destiny. The result was that I felt awkward with my relationships with people, and I lacked confidence when it came to many basic human interactions.

Doctors are often book smart but lack experience and knowledge in many aspects of life. At times, they really don't understand much about people or about how the world works. Medical training actually promotes social isolation! There were times when I would rather have been on a desert island than to have been around one more patient.

Experience is our best teacher. We need to experience other people to be good doctors. There is no way to learn how to feel comfortable around people unless you allow yourself to be around them.

All work and no play make Jack an incredibly frustrated and socially inept boy! It makes him a "kid in a candy store" when life suddenly fills him with temptation and riches.

Three Plagues: Fear, Guilt, and Second-Guessing

There are two things that I have been afraid of since becoming a doctor: one is the fear of making a mistake, and the other is how I would feel if I made a mistake or error in judgment that jeopardized someone's health. Unfortunately, I have discovered the answer to my second fear: it's called guilt.

I have sent people to surgery to have their hearts fixed by the best surgeons in the world. Some of them have died as a result of the surgery. When this happens, I feel like I sentenced that person to death. It is hard to live with the thought that someone could have lived longer if you had made a different recommendation. We try to help people as doctors, but sometimes the results aren't what we want or anticipate.

A long time ago, I recommended a valve replacement for a woman whose mitral valve was badly leaking. Her symptoms included shortness of breath, but otherwise she was not in bad shape for someone in her seventies. She was very active and wanted to lead a full life. I felt it best to repair the valve while she was stable and in relatively good health. I was certain that the risks would be greater later and that her health would be improved. So I recommended an operation.

She had multiple complications that were unavoidable and died the night of the surgery. I felt anguish when I heard of her death, and I also felt guilt because she would have been alive for a longer period of time had I treated her conservatively with medication. **I felt responsible.**

I rationalized to myself that it was just her time, that unforeseen complications can sometimes arise, and that it was just not my fault. My brain whispered, "There was just no choice." Unfortunately, there was a choice; there almost always is. All the wiggling in the world couldn't get me off my own hook.

Second-guessing didn't bring my patient back to life, nor did it make me feel any better as a doctor. This was a lesson that brought home the realization that medicine is not an exact science. Life and death decisions are made with the best information and scientific data possible, but there's no way of knowing who will make it and who won't, even in the hands of the best surgeons in the world.

If I could, I would ask my patients who didn't make it for forgiveness and pray that I make the best decisions that I can in my patients' interests in the future. But I no longer torture myself by second-guessing. I constantly reevaluate my decisions and learn from them. That is part of being a doctor. I try to ignore the armchair quarterbacks. Unfortunately, many of them are called lawyers.

Making agonizing decisions is what being a doctor is all about, and it's not for the faint of heart. The path of a healer is often uncertain and unclear:

The Path of a Healer

How do I make the unbearable
Bearable?
How can I ease his pain?
The body is but mortal.
Can I unlock its heavy chain?

Pain so agonizing pierces it thru
How can I numb flesh's pain
So severe?
How can I help him? What should I do?
My path as a healer is often unclear.

Xanax Was My Best Friend

About ten years ago, I started taking Xanax, a valium-type sedative. I took it when the pressures were high at work (which was most of the time), and it helped me through highly emotional times, including several marriages and a particularly nasty divorce. Somewhere along the way, I found myself requiring this medication at least two to three times a day in order to feel well and to function comfortably. It helped me survive the stresses and anguish of a life tormented by long hours and daily pressures.

Xanax became not only my friend; it was my best friend! It helped me remain very calm, even in stressful situations. I didn't realize until a lot later that I was actually too calm for my own good.

Some people felt that my apparent tranquility was unusual and brought this to my attention. Others just commented that my reflexes appeared slow; sometimes I was a bit slow answering my pages and at times a little late for my rounds. I thought at the time that no harm was being done, and it seemed like a fair tradeoff: a trade of panic and stress for peace and tranquility seemed like a no-brainer. Of course, I was the only one who knew about my secret friend.

One crisis led to another at work and at home, and I found myself taking extra Xanax to numb myself to the anxiety of daily events. As time went by, it took more and more Xanax to do the job, and when I didn't take it, my body reacted by becoming agitated and nervous. It was a very uncomfortable feeling. It was easier to take the medication than to combat the jitters or to come to terms with the events that were driving me crazy.

I eventually found it a lot easier to prescribe the medication for myself than to continue to go to the doctor who wrote the prescription. I did this by calling the prescription for the Xanax into the neighborhood pharmacies. The pharmacists never questioned my refills; after all, I was a doctor with a valid medical license and DEA (Drug Enforcement Agency) number. I was also extremely busy, and it was the easy way out. I knew that I had things under control. Why should I bother my doctor when I could save him the time and effort and do it myself? I wasn't worried.

At the time, I really didn't see anything wrong with any of this. I rationalized that I was doing what was necessary for my survival. I continued to take this medication for two years, and it became very much like my American Express card: I never "left home without it." I even took it with me on holidays because I liked how it made me feel, and I didn't like how I felt without it, even when I was away from work. My new friend went with me wherever I went. It was a constant companion. If I didn't take it, it reminded me very quickly who was the boss.

This drug was insidious, just like a virus, and it gained control over me before I knew what was happening. I hit rock bottom before I sought help, and I was very lucky that I didn't kill myself or hurt any of my patients. There is one whole day that is lost to my memory because I took too many pills. I vaguely remember making rounds, but that is all that I can recall. My close friends and office staff knew that I needed help, and they helped me to see that my life literally depended on it. I went to see a therapist and minister who helped rid me of the Xanax and exorcise my demons.

In retrospect, I made several errors in my assumptions that could have literally proven fatal. My first mistake was that I thought that I had things under control and that I wasn't hooked—wrong! I was in denial! The second was that I was doing what I needed to do for self-preservation; actually I was doing quite the opposite. The third mistake was that I blinded myself into thinking that what I was doing was ethical, legal, and justifiable: totally wrong and punishable! I didn't think about consequences because I was too concerned with just getting through the ordeal that had become my life.

I needed help to treat a disease that had ruled my life for several years. It took counseling and the help of my family to lead me away from a fate of self-destruction. I was weaned off the Xanax over several months by taking the advice of others and by not being my own doctor!

It took determination and will power because my body had become close buddies with this drug. I have found other ways to feel better about life since that time, and I have found better, less fickle friends.

What happened to me could happen to anyone. Substance abuse and addiction are a lot more common and subtle than most people realize. A lot of accolades and degrees hang on my walls, but all those fancy honors and diplomas didn't prevent me from a disease that is all too common among physicians.

I had a blind spot for my own problems; this is called denial:

> **"Denial is an almost universal characteristic of the disease of addiction. Denial absolves the addict of personal accountability. This distortion of the truth is an unconscious defense mechanism that protects a damaged self-esteem while allowing the underlying disease to progress. The denial system, as well as the addictive process itself, can prevent the addicted physician from wanting or even feeling the need for treatment."**[5]

Doctors frequently witness denial in their patients, but I couldn't see when it was happening to me. I went right along thinking that things were fine and dandy, and most others didn't think anything was wrong either. Superficially I was functioning reasonably well although my personal life was a shambles. I had few interpersonal relationships with my peers and few close friends. My relationship with my wife was strained, and eventually we were divorced.

Very often, addictions can be subtle and very devious. Historically this is true, as is shown in the following letter written by Professor William Osler about his observations and concerns for his friend, Professor William Stewart Halstad:

> **"The proneness to seclusion, the slight peculiarities amounting to eccentricities at times (which to his old friends in New York seemed more strange than to us) were the only outward traces of the daily battle through which this brave fellow lived for years. When we recommended him as full surgeon to the hospital in 1890, I believed, and Welch did too, that he was no longer addicted to morphia. He had worked so well and energetically that it did not seem possible that he could take the drug and do so much.**
>
> **About six months after the full position had been given, I saw him in severe chills, and this was the first information I had that he was still taking morphia. Subsequently, I had many talks about it and gained his full confidence. He had never been able to reduce the amount to less than three grains daily; on this, he could do his work comfortably and maintain his excellent physical vigor. I do not think anyone suspected him, not even Welch."[6]**

Medical societies and medical schools didn't acknowledge the problem until the past two decades. In 1973, the AMA Council on Mental Health adopted a landmark report on "The Sick Physician",[7] which recommended that state medical societies establish programs devoted to helping impaired physicians and, secondly, that the AMA adopt legislation to amend state practice acts so that treatment rather than punitive measures could be made available. Through the AMA's efforts, every state medical society now has a policy and a committee on physician impairment.

There was a relative absence of research and teaching about alcohol and drug dependence in medical schools until recently. The pervasiveness of this problem has become more apparent; therefore, it can no longer be ignored. However, there are negative attitudes still permeating the healthcare system.

Several studies have assessed the prevalence of substance abuse and dependence disorders and have found that the incidence among physicians is 10–15 percent.[8] Data from one study has shown that the lifetime rate of alcohol disorders is 13.5 percent and that the lifetime prevalence of drug abuse and dependence is 6.2 percent overall (generally higher for men than for women).[9]

Some people are addicted to work, some to sex, and some to money or power. Some people are addicted to change or to pushing the edge. Medicine is an example of a profession where an addiction to work is praised by peers and rewarded by society in general. It is extremely beneficial and almost a requirement to be a workaholic in the medical profession.

I am convinced that people don't mysteriously become transformed into workaholics when they become doctors. Medicine attracts this personality because it is demanding and rewards this behavior. What nobler purpose could there be in life than to sacrifice yourself for your fellow man (while fulfilling an inner need at the same time)? It is interesting that "compulsivity is a primary symptom of chemical dependence"[10] while it is also a common personality trait among doctors.

No one has proven that doctors have a personality trait that predisposes them to addiction. There is also no evidence that medicine preselects those with a special risk for addiction.[11]

However, it has been shown that doctors are five times more likely than the general population to take sedatives and minor tranquilizers without medical supervision[12] while self-prescribing and self-treatment with prescription drugs has been shown to be a risk factor for chemical dependence.[13] Obviously, the milieu is right for those who are at high risk.

Who is at risk for addiction? Studies have shown that certain psychological traits put one at high risk for addiction. They include passivity and self-doubt, dependency and pessimism, as well as narcissism; even a lack of religious affiliation has been associated with a higher incidence of addiction and substance abuse. A family history of drug abuse and addiction also puts one at higher risk, so it is apparent that there is a genetic predisposition to this disease.

Despite a lack of evidence to support this theory, my personal experiences suggest that medicine attracts addictive personalities, even if the addiction is nothing more serious than to work. If work can rule your life, why can't there be another dictator, possibly one that is less benign and less forgiving?

When I took Xanax, I was trying to escape pain and anesthetize myself to the unhappy reality that I didn't particularly like myself. I had low self-esteem. I became numb to my own inner turmoil and to the pain that surrounded me in the outside world. Xanax allowed me to look in the mirror with rose-colored glasses. It made me feel like I was in control of my out-of-control life. It also allowed me to deal with the seemingly endless stream of stresses that had overtaken my life without dealing with my own problems. When I took Xanax, I felt like I could cope. The white coat did the rest.

For a physician, seeing pain and suffering is a daily fact of life. It sometimes is overwhelming. There are days when I have wept because of the anguish that I have seen, and over time, the stress and pressure of the long hours take their toll. Artificial cures for the emotional stress seemed both reasonable and necessary. Coping with stress was a matter of survival. It is for all doctors.

There are also the issues of availability and the temptation of being surrounded by drugs. Prescription medications are relatively easy for a doctor to obtain. Most pharmacies honor the prescriptions that I write without question or reservation. I have never had a prescription declined. The local pharmacists know me well, and they respect me.

Drug companies send salesmen to my office to teach me about their medications. Part of their job is to provide samples for my patients (and for my own personal needs or my family's). It's also an easy access to a wide variety of drugs. Their goal, of course, is to convince me to prescribe these medications for my patients. They are salesmen, and they are simply doing their job!

It was difficult to say "no" when I was offered free Xanax from the company salesman. I didn't have enough will power to resist the temptation that was right under my nose. The salesman became an unwitting accomplice to my problem. I will discuss the topic of "**self-prescribing**" further in the next chapter.

Drug abuse is "the great-leveler," putting doctors on the street corner with prostitutes and drug dealers. But the good news is that it is a treatable disease. There are multiple components to the treatment program, and it is a "team" approach, involving a psychiatric team, a medical addiction team, and a family therapy team, among others.

State Physician Health Programs have been important in the rehabilitation process. Successful programs have identified a number of key elements to successful treatment and recovery.

"Physicians who are most successful in their recovery avoid emotions such as anger, guilt, depression, and anxiety by using Twelve Step recovery program principles. They avoid compulsive behaviors and learn to become skillful

> **in participating in important relationships (family, sponsor, spouse, parents, children, friends, etc). They also develop a profound and abiding attitude of gratitude. They learn to have open and honest communication with family members. They are regular in their attendance at AA (or other Twelve Step meetings), they communicate with their sponsors, and check out their behavior with other family members and recovering friends. These behaviors must become part of the recovering physician's routine patterns of life."[14]**

Treatment has allowed many doctors to go back to helping others. Programs of rehabilitation have been successful in recovering over 70 percent of impaired physicians. Dr. G. Douglas Talbott is a leader in this field, and I refer you to his chapter in *Principles of Addiction Medicine, Second Edition,* for more details about his success in treating physicians who are impaired by alcohol or drug abuse.

Unfortunately, negative attitudes permeate the healthcare system and the general public. People are skeptical about a doctor with "a history." That's why privacy is important, especially to a person whose livelihood depends on his reputation. Does everyone truly have a right to know if a doctor has gone through drug rehabilitation?

We need to learn how to better prevent and treat this disease and restore impaired doctors to a useful place in their families, society, and profession. I am certainly not suggesting that impaired physicians be allowed to care for patients unless they have gone through monitored treatment programs and are in compliance with state regulations.

Thank God for second chances. As a society, we are generous with forgiveness and understanding. Does your doctor deserve less understanding than anyone else? We can't sweep the problem of addiction under the rug. It exists, and it can't be ignored.

The "Natural High" of Being a Doctor

There is nothing more powerful than the "natural high" that I have experienced as a doctor. It is a satisfying feeling to help others overcome obstacles and unlock the mysteries surrounding their bodies and minds.

Sherlock Holmes must have felt a similar sense of satisfaction when he solved an intriguing murder case. Putting the final piece into a difficult puzzle gives me a feeling of exhilaration that is hard to compare to anything else that I have ever experienced. There is more involved in this "high" than just pride and ego, but positive strokes never hurt.

Cardiologists spend a large amount of time taking care of heart-attack victims. We were so very limited in what we could do for these patients just a few years ago. Nine hundred thousand people a year die from heart disease, most of them from atherosclerosis of the coronary arteries. Technology has advanced tremendously, and we now have the ability to take people to a catheterization laboratory and reopen a totally closed blood vessel with a wire, a balloon that is several millimeters in diameter, and often a stent.

It's magic that beats even The Great Houdini! When this feat is accomplished within a few hours of the onset of the heart attack, a tremendous amount of heart muscle is potentially salvaged. This often means the difference between life and death or between a severely crippled life and a life of good quality.

Being a doctor fills me with a sense of awe and wonder. When you help a human being survive a heart attack, when he might otherwise have died, it makes you thank God for making you a doctor. You feel like you are part of a miracle, a lot like seeing childbirth. In many cases, I felt like I had been a witness to a "rebirth." My patients tell me that sometimes it is a spiritual rebirth for them as well as a physical renewal.

Being a witness to these miracles fills one with the realization that God does His work through each of us every day. At times, I feel that His hand has touched my shoulder, gently guiding me as I try to help others. He has helped me make a promise to my patients that I intend to keep:

My Promise

God gave me a gift to give to you.
That's why I am here; that's what
I came to do.
It may bring happiness or sadness,
Maybe madness;
There may be nothing that I can do,
But be with you.

Tears to my eyes you bring.
Sometimes with joy you make me sing.
I promise to be with you,
For what you must go through.

To ease your suffering is God's plan.
I will do His will the best that I can.
I promise to feel for you
For what you must go through.

You are my teacher, my reason
For being.
Thank you for giving me sight
For seeing.
I promise to be there for you
For what you must go through.

Solving a mystery is one thing; saving a person's life or changing it for the better is an unforgettable moment. But sometimes all we can do is "be there."

The "magic" of being a doctor is both humbling and awe-inspiring. The most incredible feelings that doctors can experience allow them to be "reborn" along with their patients. This feeling of peace and contentment produces a natural high that is more powerful than any medicine or drug. It is a touch of heaven on earth and is difficult to find unless one is fortunate.

Sometimes I feel a little like Harry Houdini and Sherlock Holmes rolled into one. But what's so exciting is that their illusion and mystery is the reality that doctors live every day of their lives.

It isn't every day that one sees the Phoenix rise from the ashes! Being a doctor is all about appreciating and celebrating the beauty of life and, at the same time, respecting the mysteries of both life and death.

Endnotes

1. Blanchard, *The Heart of a Leader* (Tulsa: Honor Books, 1999), p. 54.
2. Brussat and Brussat, *Spiritual Rx, Prescriptions for living a Meaningful Life* (Hyperion, 2000), p.51.
3. Ibid., p. 52.
4. Larson and Koenig, "Is God Good for Your Health? The Role of Spirituality in Medical Care," *The Cleveland Clinic Journal of Medicine*, Vol. 67, No. 2, p. 83.
5. Graham and Shultz, *Principles of Addiction Medicine, Second Edition,* (American Society of Addiction Medicine, Inc., 1998, p. 1266.
6. Ibid., p. 1264.
7. Ibid., p. 1263.
8. Guadagnino, "Treating Physician Substance Abuse," *Physician News Digest*, March 1997.
9. *Principles of Addiction Medicine*, p. 1270.
10. Ibid., p. 1265.
11. Ibid.
12. Ibid., p. 1266.
13. Ibid., p. 1274.
14. Ibid., p. 1274.

CHAPTER 3

Physician, Heal Thyself?

"A man who is his own doctor has a fool for a patient."

Montague

Doctors, like a lot of their patients, often try to be their own physicians; usually they wind up making matters worse. Some of my dearest patients try to be their own doctors. This frustrates me, and I wonder why they bother to come to see me in the first place. I also know doctors who have tried to be their own doctors, including myself, and that can result in catastrophe.

It is common for medical students and residents to think that they have every illness under the sun. After all, "a little knowledge is a dangerous thing." I remember feeling my glands when I read about lymphomas and thinking that I had leukemia and a variety of cancers and infectious diseases when I read about the symptoms that they produce.

At one time or another, I have thought that I have had every disease known to man. Human nature often allows our imaginations to overtake our common sense, especially when we are tired. Fatigue makes rationality go by the wayside; all kinds of things have popped into my head when I am sleep deprived: Could I be anemic? Maybe this lump is a tumor. These were thoughts that just couldn't be ignored, and I don't consider myself a hypochondriac.

So just what is it about doctors that tends to makes us challenging and, sometimes, impossible patients?

My experience has taught me that there are several characteristics about doctors (and nurses) that make us potentially difficult patients:

- Egotism and self-confidence: After gaining experience, doctors usually feel very confident in their abilities and their knowledge. When taking care of others, this is often a plus, but it can also be detrimental when it turns into, "I really don't need help figuring this problem out," or, "I know as much as they do about what's wrong with me."
- Independence: "I really don't want anyone else telling me what to do about my own problems," and "I'll get around to it; just get off my back!" "I really don't need that test or medication anyway" is a common refrain. Doctors, by and large, are independent creatures, and it is a hard habit to break.
- Compulsiveness and a controlling nature: "I'm going to do this my way" and "I'll decide which tests are important." Sometimes this also turns into: "I know how expensive that test is, and I'm just not going to pay that kind of money! After all, they should give me a discount because I am a physician. I deserve free care from my associates!" Most doctors don't ask for professional courtesy because it is an unspoken rule to help your colleagues.

- The temptation to self-prescribe: Most doctors don't want to go to another doctor to prescribe a "simple" antihistamine or antibiotic. This is due to several personality traits that I am describing in this section and is one of the primary reasons why doctors are dangerous to themselves (and sometimes their families). It is a primary reason why doctors make difficult patients. I will talk more about this in the next section because it deserves a lot more discussion.
- Knowing too little and too much: Doctors know just enough to be dangerous and too little to be able to assess our own needs. None of us can be objective about our problems, can we? Doctors are no exception! I've seen enough to be dangerous to my own health: "I hope they don't make a mistake" or "I've seen that complication before. I hope it doesn't happen to me." I've read about and seen mistakes and complications that can injure my own health just by knowing about them. Unfortunately, doctors have too much and also too little information, and this makes us our own worst enemies.
- Time constraints and pressures of the job: Doctors are just too busy taking care of others to take care of themselves. Stress is a major factor in the self-administration of drugs of abuse as well.[1] A lot of doctors think that they are indispensable (see under "ego" earlier); this is often a rationalization that allows us to avoid situations that are unpleasant, such as taking care of that dental exam, pelvic exam, or colonoscopy. Doctors are trained to be caregivers, and we often have a hard time looking at our own needs and sometimes the needs of our families. We have a hard time being caretakers. Recently, a pediatrics nurse whose son committed suicide lamented, "I was able to take care of everyone else's children but my own."
- Murphy's Law: Bad things happen to good people, even doctors! If something is going to go wrong, it is often

with the people that we know, especially fellow healthcare workers.

Many of these tendencies go with the territory of being a healthcare professional. I've often dreaded taking care of fellow physicians and nurses because my work is doubled trying to get them to stop diagnosing and treating themselves. On the other hand, it is an honor when a doctor or nurse asks me to take care of him or her. If someone who knows medicine thinks that you're good enough, that says a lot!

An addendum is important here. I have taken care of doctors who are wonderful patients and patients who are less than wonderful doctors.

Self-Prescribing—The Wolf Guarding the Henhouse

Self-prescribing is very common among doctors and nurses for a number of reasons: it is easy, for the most part legal, and saves time, effort, and sometimes money if free samples are available.

Drug company "sales reps" place sample packets and stock bottles of medications in a special closet in doctors' offices every day. These drugs are intended to be samples for patients starting on new prescriptions—i.e., starter kits for antihypertensives and diabetics—and they are also for those who can't afford to buy them. Most offices have drug closets like my own for such medicines. They are usually unlocked but certainly not open to the public.

Controlled substances are generally placed in a separate area under lock and key. Even the Viagra is locked up because it disappears so quickly! Of course, as the doctor in the office, I have a key. I could take any one of a number of antihistamines, anti-inflammatory drugs, or a variety of uncontrolled medications home for myself or for my family without being accountable to anyone. The doctor and his staff have discretionary power over how the drugs in their possession are dispersed.

For many years, doctors have been given samples of sedatives like Xanax. To this day, drug companies still freely provide samples of hypnotics or sleep medicines that can't be bought over the counter. Other controlled drugs are not hard to obtain from drug companies by special request.

Prescriptions written by doctors usually go to the local drug store. Pharmacies will almost never say no to a prescription written by a physician as long as the DEA number is given over the phone or is written on the prescription. Over the years, I have written my own refills for antibiotics, sedatives, and even pain pills that are "controlled" substances without being questioned.

Local pharmacists have a loyalty to fellow healthcare professionals, and it is also just good business not to upset local physicians. Pharmacists generally want to keep doctors happy because of the good will they provide to their patients. It is hard to say "no" when the doctor calls asking for help.

Over the years, I have definitely crossed an ethical line even if I didn't do anything that is technically illegal. Over-the-counter (OTC) medicines are offered to the public because they are generally felt to be safe. Should doctors be any different? Are pharmacists and drug-company sales representatives silent accomplices to the larger problem of physician drug abuse? Should doctors be allowed to self-prescribe any controlled substances at all?

The reality is that doctors do self-prescribe. No one ever told me that I couldn't prescribe Xanax for myself, and no pharmacist ever refused my written or verbal requests for any drug other than for those requiring "triplicate" written forms. Triplicate forms are used for the most highly regulated drugs such as morphine and amphetamines. Many narcotics, however, do not require triplicate forms, i.e., Darvocet and

Vicodin. I can "call in" (phone the pharmacist) and get refills for these without a problem.

The regulations that do exist are poor and ineffective, and it is therefore very easy for doctors to obtain drugs and treat themselves. The ramifications of this practice are obvious, not only to a doctor's physical and mental health but to his professional health as well.

Many doctors are not able to resist the temptation to treat themselves. Self-prescribing is quick, easy, and perhaps the main reason why doctors make the worst patients and why they also present the most challenging treatment problems. Vaillant (1992) has identified self-prescribing and self-treatment with prescription drugs as a risk factor for chemical dependence,[2] and Hughes and colleagues (1992) found that physicians were more likely than their non-physician counterparts to take sedatives and minor tranquilizers without medical supervision.[3]

We really have left the "wolf guarding the henhouse," or rather the drug cabinet. But the wolf is often a tired and stressed-out creature who may give into temptation when he feels cornered and hungry. Stress is a factor in addiction, and it makes a doctor more prone to the problems that I have discussed.

Reread "**Xanax Was My Best Friend**" in Chapter 2 if there are any doubts in your mind about how easily self-medicating and addiction can occur. Tighter controls are necessary to protect both the patients from their doctors and the doctors from themselves. Finding ways to combat stress and fatigue are important not only for the profession as a whole but also for the individual whose job it is to help others manage their stress and health problems.

The "Curbside" Consult

It's commonplace for a nurse or a doctor to see another healthcare professional in the hallway at the hospital, or even on the street, and ask for an opinion about his or her medical problems. This is called "the curbside consult" and is appropriately named because this discussion tends to occur in the middle of the busy traffic of the day and can easily lead to an awful accident. The curbside consult is one way to get advice without going through the formality of an office consultation, which can be too costly, bothersome, and too time consuming.

It can also be a detour around the path to good medical care. It is a shortcut that is nerve-wracking and unfair to the person on the receiving end and that can lead to errors in communication and misunderstandings. The shortcut often leads to obstacles and hazards that could have been prevented by going the correct route.

Detours and shortcuts generally sabotage a doctor's care. I have tried to avoid these detours like the plague, but all too often, I have sometimes found myself discussing my own problems with colleagues in the hallways. Generally, other doctors are gracious and listen, but deep down they are probably thinking that they would rather I do things correctly and see them in their offices where they can conduct proper history and physical examinations prior to giving me their recommendations. Anything less is unacceptable for our patients, and it should be for us, too, despite the fact that we are doctors.

I recently took care of a nurse who was told casually by a doctor that she worked with that there was no cause for alarm regarding her chest pains. She continued to have pain and eventually came to see me in my office. I discovered a 99 percent blockage in a major artery in her heart that was about to cause a major heart attack. Her curbside consult almost led to an early demise. The words that she told me echoed in my mind: "There's nothing wrong; you're a young nurse, probably too tired, and besides, you're not the right sex to have a heart attack anyway!"

It's a fact that women are "written off" by doctors as being neurotic or hormonal when they often have real heart disease or other organic illness. This problem is especially true when the women are nurses or healthcare professionals. Doctors have no choice but to take everyone, including themselves, seriously; that means getting ourselves proper care that cannot be properly delivered via a curbside consult.

Taking care of fellow physicians sometimes leads to subtle changes in the way that one normally treats patients. To avoid making mistakes, sometimes more tests are ordered than usual, and to avoid ringing up the cash register, some tests are avoided or ignored that otherwise would have been done. Sometimes there is a little arm-twisting that goes on such as, "Do you really think I need this test? I really don't think I have any major problems."

I love it when the doctor or nurse/patient says to me, "Just do what you normally do. Don't make any exceptions to the rules!"

This tongue twister addresses the challenges of "doctoring doctors":

"If a doctor is doctoring a doctor
Does the doctor doing the doctoring
Doctor the doctor being doctored
The way the doctor being doctored
Wants to be doctored,
Or does the doctor doctoring the doctor
Doctor the doctor being doctored
The way the doctoring doctor usually doctors?"[4]

Several points are important to remember when a doctor takes care of another doctor or his or her family:

- It is better not to take care of other physicians if it is likely to provoke an excessive degree of anxiety. It is possible to feel that your competence will be scrutinized more than usual. The resulting tension may lead to indecisive actions.[5]
- A doctor should not perform the history and physical any differently for other doctors than he does for his regular patients. It is important not to avoid asking personal questions. Intimate parts of the exam should not be omitted, such as a rectal or pelvic exam.
- "Many physicians tend to make incorrect self-diagnoses with absolute certainty, particularly in fields other than their own."[6] It is important to remember that the physician/patient is anxious about his or her diagnosis, and it is important to take his or her feelings seriously.
- The nature of the relationship needs to be clarified as early as possible. It is important to make the physician/patient aware that he or she will be treated like any other patient and not like a "VIP." Confidentiality must be handled as it would in any other doctor-patient relationship. Financial arrangements should also be discussed early in the relationship. Sometimes the treating physician won't charge at all or will take what insurance will pay and write off the rest (insurance-only billing). The expectations of the physician/patient may not be the same as those of the treating doctor. "Professional courtesy" sometimes has a different meaning to different people and may not always mean free care.
- It is important to avoid overly close empathy or sympathy. "Modifying routines to save the patient time, trouble, and money may result in poor medical care."[7]

An overly close relationship may inhibit the role reversal that is necessary for a doctor to become a patient.

- Don't assume that doctors know about their diseases and about the medications that they are being asked to take. It is important not to make assumptions about a doctor's knowledge, especially when his problems are outside his field of expertise. The treating physician needs to thoroughly discuss the diagnosis and treatment plan as he would with any other patient.

"To be known as a "doctor's doctor" is both an accolade and a challenge."[8] A psychiatrist-friend warned me: "As patients, doctors can be a tough nut to crack." Over the years, I have come to learn that taking care of doctors can be both frustrating and rewarding.

I found out from first-hand experience that it is tough to be both a doctor and a patient. Fate made the decision for me. I was forced to learn what it was like to get a "taste of my own medicine."

Getting a Taste of My Own Medicine

"I'd rather be a hammer than a nail....Yes, I would, if I only could, I surely would."

"El Condor Pasa (If I Could)," Simon and Garfunkel

It was a typical late night in Ben Taub's I.C.U. (intensive care unit). I was on call and had admitted several critically ill patients. Sleep was an oasis in the desert. It was 3 A.M. when a drug addict rolled in through the door. He was comatose from an overdose of an unknown drug, and he was seizing and needed help with ventilating his lungs.

Mr. D.A. (drug addict) couldn't get enough oxygen to the vital organs of his body because his lungs weren't working properly. It was my job to stabilize my patient and try to prevent complications until his kidneys and liver could excrete the drugs that were in his system, while protecting his vital organs from irreversible damage.

My job as an intern was to "draw" blood on my patients, especially those who were critically ill. Ben Taub had lab techs, but at 3 A.M., the staff was thin, and it could take hours to draw the lab tests and get the results that I desperately needed. Mr. D.A. was critically ill and couldn't afford to wait for the techs to get there to draw the blood for his very important tests.

Minutes were precious in the I.C.U. Lives were at stake, and I felt intense pressure during my nights on call to get things done promptly and efficiently. This was not only for my patients' sakes but also to save my own hide and avoid being the sacrificial lamb at morning report. As you probably realized while reading Chapter 1, the stress of working in the I.C.U. is incredible.

Taking the blood from Mr. D.A.'s arm went uneventfully. I had become very adept at finding veins with the touch of my finger and a needle. Generally, I stuck needles into about twenty-five veins during an average day at work.

The next step was to put the blood into a tube called a vacutainer, which is a glass test tube fitted with a rubber stopper that sucks the blood from the syringe into the tube by virtue of its vacuum. The vacutainer containing the blood specimen was then sent to the lab for analysis.

Dead tired and in a hurry, I missed the vacutainer with the syringe needle. I felt the stabbing pain in my finger instantly. It was brief but alerted me quickly to what I had done. I remember thinking to myself: "What a nuisance! I really don't have time for this." I quickly withdrew the needle from my finger, threw it out in a special "sharps container," and finished my job of transferring the blood to the lab for final processing.

At that time, there was no AIDS epidemic, and there were no needle precautions other than, of course, "being careful." A half hour after sending Mr. D.A.'s specimens to the lab, I washed my hands, filled out the appropriate incident report forms, and received a shot of gamma globulin, the standard treatment for this sort of accident.

At the time, I was worried more about my patient than about myself. It was not the first time that I had stuck myself, but it was the deepest stick that I had sustained with a dirty needle. I felt that it was more of a nuisance than anything else and came with the territory of being a doctor. I don't even remember drawing blood work to see if the patient had liver abnormalities suggesting hepatitis, a viral infection of the liver that could be transferred by needle stick.

I started feeling increased fatigue within the next few months but otherwise felt normal. For an intern, fatigue is a way of life, so this really didn't faze me or give me any cause for concern. I didn't go to see a doctor because I was too busy and couldn't take the time for "trivial" problems. Eventually, when I continued to feel tired, I had blood drawn in the lab to look for possible etiologies of my chronic fatigue.

The results surprised me. My liver enzymes were mildly abnormal. "No big deal, probably just a mild inflammation from working too hard and not getting enough rest," I said to myself. I attributed it to stress and to drinking some alcohol with my friends on my rare nights off.

The fatigue continued and increased, and six months later, the enzymes were still elevated. I finally went to see a liver specialist who did more blood work in order to find out if I had hepatitis A or B. Both came back negative, and I was relieved, thinking that this would all go away and was only a bad dream.

My doctor's diagnosis was "Non A, Non B Hepatitis." Very little was known about this disease, but he didn't seem to be overly worried, so I wasn't either. The virus had inadvertently entered my bloodstream when I stuck myself with the contaminated needle.

A liver biopsy was performed that showed an essentially normal liver, so I again went about my usual routine of hard work, little sleep, and eating hamburgers and snacks on the run. That's the typical life of most interns, and not a very healthy lifestyle at that. I still sometimes went to the neighborhood bars with my fellow interns when we got off from work. This was where we unwound and got away from it all.

This form of hepatitis was felt to be benign at that time, so no treatment or further tests were recommended. I monitored my lab work intermittently for years and was reassured by colleagues that, although not much was known about this disease, there was probably not much cause for alarm or concern.

In the nineties, more became known about this virus that became labeled Hepatitis C (HCV). The symptoms of HCV are subtle, and the fatigue that it causes can be easily confused with normal fatigue, as had been done in my case. Meanwhile, the virus causes its silent damage.

HCV results in chronic hepatitis in 80 percent of patients and cirrhosis in 20 to 35 percent. It is a slowly progressive disease that is the leading cause of liver transplantation and also is strongly associated with the development of liver cancer. It is now known that alcohol speeds the progression of the disease and makes its treatment less effective. Needless to say, I have said goodbye to the bars.

It has taken me years to discover that I have a potentially deadly invader in my system. I have undergone four liver biopsies over twenty-two years, which have shown slow progression of the disease. Fatigue is my frequent partner, but I still feel that a lot of it is due to the hard and grueling work of being a doctor.

I have flashbacks of the needle stick that remind me of the insidious virus that is in my system, a virus that was put inside my body by my own carelessness and by the recklessness of someone that I never knew. I can still feel and see the dirty needle embedding itself in my skin and now realize how life can change in a fraction of an instant. By the way, Mr. D.A. was discharged from the hospital and was eventually readmitted with a fatal overdose of heroin a few months after my accident.

Since my diagnosis, I have undergone two rounds of therapy with interferon, a drug also used to treat both cancer and hepatitis, and a second drug called ribaviron. Both treatments yielded only temporary remissions with normalization of my liver enzymes and a decrease in my viral load (a blood test that measures the amount of virus in the blood is called HCV PCR).

Unfortunately, the enzyme levels rebounded after the yearlong treatment was finished. I quickly discovered how my patients must feel when they have their hopes for a cure dashed after experiencing an initially successful treatment.

Both courses of treatment produced side effects that were significant enough to make it a challenge to get through the day. I suffered from extreme fatigue, weight loss of twenty pounds, fever, and even depression.

My hair thinned out, even more than usual for my age, but came back later. I continued to work, taking catnaps in between patients to make it through the day. The syringes filled with interferon delivered both medicine and hope through a sliver of steel that became:

My Painful Friend

I held above my thigh
A shiny piece of steel,
Poised in mid-air
My fate to seal.

As it pierces my flesh,
My eyes close, a wince crosses
My face,
A unique reminder
Of my past mistakes.

A painful friend that makes me feel
Well and ill,
Giving my body fatigue and chills,
I must accept it without fear
Or remorse,
As a messenger of hope
From a higher source.

So far this pesky organism has outsmarted everything that I have thrown in its path. Fortunately, the treatments that I took have helped to cure about half the people with HCV and have given them a new lease on life. Subsequently, the FDA approved this experimental protocol for the treatment of patients with HCV.

It felt good to have taken part in a study that had helped other people, but I had more selfish motivations. I settled for the fact that the treatments had bought me some more time by temporarily reducing the virus in my system and delaying its progression, but I was obviously disappointed that the treatments didn't cure me.

I felt like I was on a roller-coaster ride and someone else was in control of the ups and downs in my life. I just knew that I was the one who was living the nightmare, and I definitely was grasping for ways to take control of the situation.

Numerous emotions have surrounded the virus that has become my constant companion for the past twenty years. Although contracting a disease like HCV is an occupational hazard for everyone in the medical profession, this thought hasn't helped me feel better about the situation that I have found myself in.

I can now understand the anger of AIDS patients who contracted this lethal disease through the promiscuity of others. At the same time that I am angry, I am thankful that I didn't contract AIDS. I was just doing my job to the best of my ability. Fatigue caused me to be careless, but **the simple truth is that I just didn't think that this could happen to me**.

Having a chronic illness has changed how I view both life and death. I have learned to be thankful for each and every day that I am alive and to be optimistic for what the future holds. When I talk to my patients, I try to remember my own fears and frustrations. I try to remember how important it is to be compassionate and to have things explained in a way that is understandable and empathetic.

I try to remember that my patients have their own fears, just as I have mine, and that they are groping for answers that I sometimes just don't have, no matter how hard I try.

One of the important lessons that I have learned as a patient is that no one cares about my own particular situation as much as I do. I have learned the importance of becoming proactive in one's care. I have scoured the Internet and researched scores of medical journals, searching for opinions and ways to deal with my illness. If I'm not going to work hard on my own behalf, then how can I expect others to help?

As with certain other diseases, there is a "stigma" associated with hepatitis. People are generally afraid of the unknown, and a lot is not known about this illness.

Public awareness is crucial because Hepatitis C has reached epidemic proportions, and we are just seeing the tip of the iceberg. Many people are afraid to be around someone with Hepatitis C. There is a lack of understanding about this disease, and with this lack of understanding comes distrust and avoidance. Education of the public is critically important, but I had to start by educating myself first.

At times, my illness has led to feelings of isolation, fear, and anger. No one else can fight my fight for me. But I understand the importance and necessity of having the support of friends and family.

I have joined a local support group of fellow patients with HCV. When I am at these meetings, I make it very clear that I am there as a patient and not as a doctor. We are all in this large boat together, and we need to make it home in the storm. We are stronger together than we are apart.

Until I got sick with HCV, I never really knew what my patients went through just to cope with their illnesses. Previously, I had considered proactive patients to be pests and nuisances. I barely tolerated them, and, frankly, they annoyed me. I had to learn what it felt like to lose control before I could see the importance and necessity of taking control of my own destiny. I had to "walk the walk" before I could truly walk side by side with my patients.

God has given me the powerful realization that He is there to help us deal with the pain and frustrations of our afflictions. I have prayed to Him for guidance as a human being, not as someone with a title or fancy initials attached to his name. A hepatitis virus doesn't discriminate between a doctor and a drug addict. Certainly I shouldn't expect God to treat me any differently from any other living creature just because I wear a white coat.

I have discovered that "attitude" can be a valuable friend or foe in the healing process. I have cared for patients on a daily basis who get better or worse as their frames of mind dictate.

The adage "mind over matter" is best exemplified by the "placebo effect," which is when a patient feels better because he thinks he is being treated with an effective medication rather than a sugar pill. When I am tired, my mind plays tricks on me. Recognizing this, I try to keep a positive attitude because it is crucial for my health and mental well-being. Being a doctor doesn't make me any less susceptible than the rest of the world to depression and pessimism.

I have experienced the anxiety and fears associated with illness, and I've realized that they are powerful enough to control my life if I give them the opportunity. It's important to "live" life and not dwell on the past or on the negatives. It's also important to keep a sense of humor and think positively, to view the glass as "half full rather than half empty." The "power of positive thinking" is real!

I have indulged myself in pity parties, and I can hold a heck'uva good one! It's awfully easy to feel sorry for yourself when you feel that you've been dealt a bad hand. But then the thought hits me: "How can I feel sorry for myself when I take care of patients in their thirties and forties who can't walk across the room without getting chest pain?" Self-indulgence won't help me get well, and it certainly won't make me feel better physically or mentally, at least not in the long run.

Both the disease and its treatment have affected me emotionally. Interferon is known for causing depression, and it's not uncommon for its recipients to require antidepressants throughout the treatment period. I suffered through sleepless nights and became depressed while taking this drug.

Counseling and medication helped me get through the tough times. I'm not ashamed of this, but I am ashamed that I waited so long before admitting that I needed help. Depression was something for other people, not for me! Doctors don't have the time for such nuisances. We are here to take care of other people's problems. There is no time for our own!

When it comes to my own medical problems, I have learned that it is necessary to think not as a doctor but as a human being. I remind myself constantly not to try to outsmart my own caregivers, or myself, for that matter. Deep down, I know that I can't be emotionally objective enough to treat my own problems. Placing my trust in others was an absolutely necessary first step. My illness was one problem that I had to admit that I couldn't solve by myself.

It's important to be proactive, but I have discovered that I need to avoid fighting for control with my own doctor. Control is a hard thing for a lot of doctors to relinquish. Most of us are so "anal!"

I also know that **I have just enough knowledge to be dangerous**. I have had to learn to be the student, not the teacher. The roles had to be reversed.

Being on the receiving end of the needle means more than just feeling the pain piercing through your flesh. I had to allow myself to learn from others and become accustomed to a different way of thinking. I was forced to ask myself: "How would I want my patient to react in this situation?" Should the expectations that I have of myself be any different than the expectations that I have of my own patients? The answer was a resounding "**No**!"

My patients have exemplified incredible courage, grace, and even humor in the face of terrible pain and suffering and often against insurmountable odds. I am ashamed to be anything less while dealing with my own problems. They are my examples and role models, and now I have become their student.

When I think about the agony and the seeming "unfairness of life" that I have seen in my patients, I realize that my own problems are neither that terrible nor unfair. Being both doctor and patient has helped me to discover a different perspective on things.

On the other hand, I have had the opportunity as a doctor to see people die of cirrhosis, and it's not a pretty sight. It's downright scary! Recently I took care of a patient with Hepatitis C who was admitted with a heart attack. He was "encephalopathic," meaning that he didn't know where he was or what year it was. His mind was disoriented due to the high ammonia levels caused by his liver disease. He also started to bleed through his gastrointestinal tract from esophageal varices caused by cirrhosis.

I knew that he was dying from the disease that I myself was carrying, and the experience made me realize that I would do anything to avoid his fate! Every time that I visited his room, it brought me back to a reality that I didn't particularly want to think about. Deep down in my gut, I was afraid to look. But my profession gave me no alternative.

The common denominator and the great equalizer is that we are all patients at some points in our lives and that eventually we all will meet the same common destiny. I realize that I can become ill as easily as my patients. My patients sometimes tease me that doctors aren't allowed to get sick or injured; they shouldn't have common ailments. I know that they are being playful. It is reassuring to them to know that their doctor is human and that my own illness gives me the opportunity to understand what they are going through.

Being a patient has made me realize that **I am not indispensable**. When I'm feeling sick and can't work, there are others who can mind the store. Again, it's a matter of giving up control (and my compulsiveness). I've also learned to be kinder to myself and to rethink my priorities in life. I have had to reassess what is really important to me.

All doctors should be on the receiving end of the needle at one time or another. That doesn't mean that they need to get some horrible disease or go through major surgery to understand the plights of others.

But being a patient does help a doctor to be empathetic for what others are experiencing and feeling. I now ask myself: "How would it feel to be told what I am being told or to be treated the way I am being treated?" The answers are not found in any textbook. I have tried to put myself in my patients' minds.

Thus far, the "unwanted house guest" in my body has refused to surrender to my best efforts. But I have also refused to surrender to it as well. It does its work in stealth and hides from view. It's a pest, a predator, a parasite, and a chameleon that has "chutzpah." It changes shape almost at will. At times, I feel like Luke Skywalker summoning "the force" to battle against Darth Vader and "the dark side."

I've learned from first-hand experience that medicine does not have all the answers. I am looking outside the realm of conventional medicine, not out of desperation but because I realize that doctors are human. I have learned a number of lessons from the other life force that exists within my body. It has taught me ways to think and feel that have made me a better person as well as a better doctor.

I also have learned the importance of prayer, faith, and hope. And I have learned the importance of chasing my dreams from:

My Enemy Within

Tiny beast and predator
Stalking its prey silently
Turned my life into a nightmare,
And became a formidable adversary.
Eating away at each living cell,
Multiplying faster and faster,
Changing its shape at will,
Can I thwart this tiny chameleon
Who flaunts its power still?

A villain with many disguises and names,
Pest and parasite are a few,
Uninvited houseguest who I blame

And admire
For its guile and "chutzpah" too!

This micron-sized stalker to whom I've
Fallen prey
Liberates and elevates me
To the need to pray
And to kneel,
And allows me the pain of others to feel.

This life within a life
Has changed mine forever
For the better and for the worse.
It makes me stronger thru' my strife.
It is both a blessing and a curse.

Endnotes

1. Angres and Talbott, *Healing the Healer, The Addicted Physician* (Madison, Connecticut, Psychosocial Press, 1998), p. 97.
2. Graham and Shultz, *The Principles of Addiction Medicine, Second Edition* (American Society of Addiction Medicine, Inc., 1998) p. 1265.
3. Ibid.
4. Lipsitt, "Letter to the Editor," *Journal of the American Medical Association*, Vol. 281, No. 12, March 31, 1999. Also see Lipsitt, "The Doctor as Patient," *Psychiatric Opinion*, 1975, 12:20–25.
5. Schneck, "Doctoring Doctors and their Families," *Journal of the American Medical Association*, Vol. 280, 2039–042.
6. Ibid.
7. Ibid.
8. Ibid.

CHAPTER 4

Used and Abused, Audited and Sued

"Getting Away From It All"

One of my favorite pictures is of a duck surrounded by four alligators. The duck is blissfully sleeping on a beach unaware that anything is threatening him. Four alligators are waiting to pounce on their prey from all angles while the duck is totally unaware of his predators. This painting is entitled, "Getting Away From It All" and was painted in 1987 by the renowned artist Michael Bedard. I have it hanging in my office where I can look at it daily for comic relief. Bedard's work makes me laugh at the harsh reality of being a doctor.

You see, I can relate to that poor duck. All he wants to do is bask in the sun. He is blissfully unaware of the threats that surround him. Being totally naïve, the duck just wants to enjoy life, go about his business, and remain blissfully ignorant.

It took me years to know the names of these four alligators. They are the personal injury and divorce lawyers (commonly known as **Liti-Gators**), the managed-care insurance industry, the personal space invaders, and, finally, the fourth alligator represents the borrowers and speculators who want to invest or borrow my money for their purposes. The odds are that most doctors will eventually deal with at least one of the four alligators along the way. They are somewhat like the flu: they make you sick to your stomach, their effects usually last more than twenty-four hours, and they leave you feeling drained and miserable.

I have come to realize that there is a fifth alligator, that isn't in the picture; it works behind the scenes. He is the "instigator alligator," and his alias is "false expectations." He is the real troublemaker of the group and is dangerous because he isn't as visible as his counterparts and often does their "dirty work."

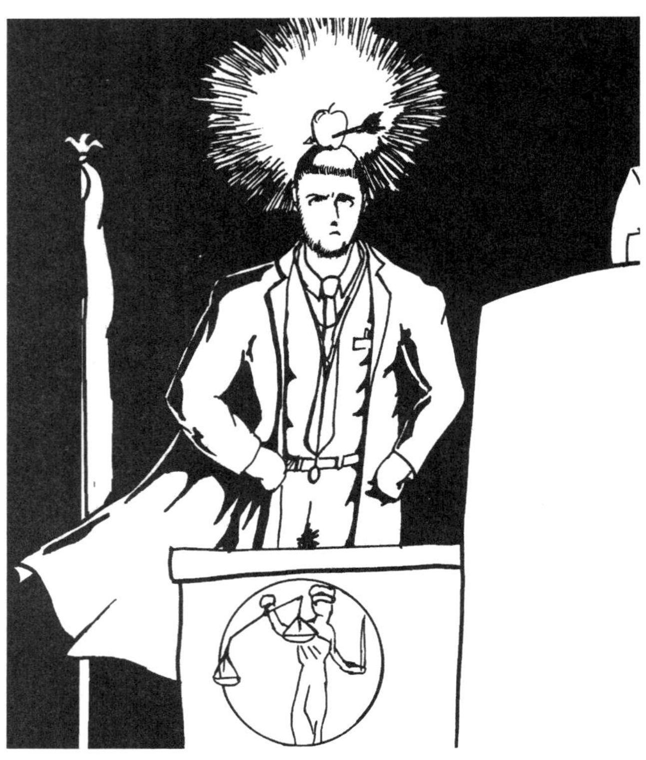

An Apple a day?

Mom, Apple Pie, and...Attorney's Fees

Q: "What do you call fifty lawyers stranded on a deserted island?"

A: "A good start."

Author Unknown; Most Likely a Doctor

Let's set the record straight, please: lawyers are **not** a doctor's worst enemy. When it comes to malpractice suits, doctors are their own worst nightmares! Sure, lawyers are ready to pounce on doctors who make mistakes; but that is their living. Can you blame them for doing their job, especially when cases are gift-wrapped and handed to them by the medical profession?

Let's face it! We have created a society that is run and virtually controlled by attorneys, and the result has been an endless sea of litigation that has taken on epidemic proportions.

Lawyer-politicians make up the rules, and as a result, dockets are overflowing with lawsuits. What we have created is as American as Mom, apple pie, and...of course, The World Wrestling Federation's pay-per-view on T.V. It's no-holds-barred, a doctor's worst nightmare, and an attorney's pot at the end of the rainbow. "Stone Cold," you're no match for "Judge Judy." She'll pin you to the courtroom floor for the count of three every time!

First, let me share some information about how our system of jurisprudence works when it comes to medical malpractice. Attorneys generally spend a lot of time interviewing their clients before they decide whether "it pays" to take on a suit and whether a suit is valid.

About one-third of malpractice cases that are screened are potential lawsuits. If a case appears to fit the legal and economic criteria of the firm, then medical records are requested from the doctor and the hospital. This may take months and costs the firm money, time, and a lot of effort.

The firm's financial investment starts here as the records often are thousands of pages and sometimes difficult to decipher (especially the doctor's). These records are reviewed by members of the firm as to their potential for litigation. If the chart passes this stage of screening, it is sent to an expert witness who is often a physician.

The expert witness, who I will henceforth refer to as "the hired gun," has the job of giving medical input as to whether malpractice was committed by the doctor or hospital staff.

The "hired gun" is often paid an hourly wage, which, in my experience, is what the doctor requests. Generally, the expert states his or her position as to whether the defendant has practiced in a way that conforms to the standard medical care for the community. Of course, this opinion is obviously unbiased!

The decision to litigate is generally based on a "standard of care," but there are a lot of other factors that lawyers consider, such as negligence, causation, and damages. In large firms, about one out of fifteen cases are accepted as meeting these legal criteria. A case also must pass a financial screening because it is not inexpensive to litigate.

Attorneys must count on winning a big settlement that will allow them to write off this overhead cost in the process. It's a gamble, one that I would compare to "Russian Roulette."

In today's managed-care market, doctors are looking more than ever for ways to supplement their income. Many of them are also running scared because of the constant fear of litigation and would love to befriend attorneys by working with them rather than against them. After all, some think that "if you can't beat 'em, join 'em!"

Being an expert witness is a way of making a few extra bucks as long as you don't mind eating your own kind for lunch and getting a reputation as a "bottom-feeder." Lawyers generally pay better than Medicare and managed care, and let's face it, a lot of people will sell their souls for money.

The first time that I was a plaintiff's witness also turned out to be my last. The experience made me feel like a traitor, and I didn't enjoy being grilled like a hamburger in court. It wasn't worth the money, even though I was asked to name my own hourly price. I also learned that it is not very smart to get a reputation as an expert witness against doctors who are practicing in nearby communities and who may someday help to pay your bills.

Why is the medical profession a prime target for both legitimate and frivolous lawsuits? A major reason is that doctors are "deep pockets" because of the huge amount of malpractice insurance that they must carry in order to practice medicine in today's world.

Many insurance companies will not contract with doctors unless they carry at least one million dollars of coverage per event and three million total aggregate over a year (meaning a total of three million for the entire year). Most hospitals require doctors to carry malpractice insurance in order to maintain staff privileges.

Another reason for the explosion of lawsuits is the history of large settlements that have been awarded by juries in the past. Lawyers know the limits of a doctor's coverage when they decide to accept a case. They know who the "deep pockets" are before deciding whether filing a lawsuit is cost effective.

A recent article in *Medical Economics* underscores the importance of economics in a firm's decision to pursue litigation. A plaintiff's attorney tells the truth about the way most firms think in terms of dollars and cents:

"The first thing we need to assess is the dollar value of the damage. If there's no damage, then there's no case for us, no matter how badly the doctor may have screwed up. I could be more compassionate about it, but that's the real basis for our decision: You establish the damages first, then the liability.…Because of our time investment and costs, we really can't consider a case unless we expect a payoff of at least $200,000 in damages, and even that's really not enough. If we end up taking a case to trial, we're probably going to spend $20,000 to $30,000 or more. So we have to make a business decision: Are the potential damages worth the time and expense we'll have to invest to win? If the damage is, say, $50,000, that may be a big deal for many people, but it's not enough to make the case worthwhile for us. So we'll turn it down."[1]

The clients who are rejected get the attorneys who are in *The Yellow Pages*! Contingency fees make it easier for clients to obtain attorneys, but they are a gamble for the attorneys, one that potentially allows them to make more money off a case than their clients. Often 40 percent of the first $150,000 and a third of the remainder of the settlement goes to the attorney with the client getting the rest after out-of-pocket expenses are paid.

Lawyers often use a "shotgun" approach, naming every physician who is involved in the case as a defendant, and then sorting out the guilty from the innocent later. Doctors are often "guilty by association." If enough mud is slung against a wall, some of it might stick!

Doctors who are innocent of any wrongdoing often get named as a defendant along with everyone else whose name is on the chart. I pray that my name isn't mentioned anywhere in a chart that is being subpoenaed because I can count on being sued if it is, whether I am guilty or not.

Then there is the matter of public perception. The medical profession is still considered by the public to be a rich profession that too often takes advantage of "John Q. Citizen." This perception, although it is usually inaccurate, makes it easy for juries to award settlements to those who are perceived as victims, especially to someone who is poor, crippled, or unemployed due to a disability.

Doctors are in a great position to help people, but they also are in a perfect position to do quite a bit of harm. They can turn from hero to scapegoat in literally a heartbeat.

Everything that a doctor does involves taking "risks," from minor operations to complicated brain surgery.

A problem may be mishandled or mistreated in numerous ways. Doctors may create bad outcomes by using poor technique, but sometimes things just go wrong without any obvious wrongdoing. I have found that "Murphy's Law" is alive and well in everyone's life, including my own. I can treat two people with identical illnesses almost exactly alike, and the outcomes will be totally different.

Usually the fate of my patients is out of my hands, even if I do everything "by the book." Unfortunately, doing everything "right" or "to the best of my abilities" doesn't always avert a lawsuit, especially if the patient or family has negative feelings towards me, or if they are angry. Sometimes it doesn't take a lot to make anxious people angry or hostile. We'll talk more about that later.

A good example of a potential land mine for a doctor is what is called medical record "documentation." Documentation includes everything from doctors' and nurses' notes to orders and lab reports. Everything on the chart is a part of a patient's medical record. It is where doctors identify and justify everything that they do.

If adequate documentation is missing from the medical record, then a doctor is as guilty in a court of law as if he physically committed malpractice. This may be an implied guilt of omission rather than one of commission. Because of this standard, a doctor can be judged guilty if the records are missing important information or were just sloppy or illegible. A doctor is, unfortunately, "guilty unless proven innocent" by the factual information on the chart.

Sloppy charting is what condemns most doctors and makes them guilty. Unless it was charted, it wasn't done, period! Sounds like there was a method to the madness back in medical training when our mentors were sticklers about everything that we wrote in our charts.

Careful documentation is also important in patient care. Consulting doctors involved in a case need to be able to understand what is being done for the patient and know what other doctors are thinking and doing. Doctors learn that it is as necessary to spend as much time accurately keeping medical records as they do physically taking care of their patients. The two go hand in hand, by necessity.

The S.O.A.P. system (Subjective information as to how the patient feels; Objective data entry such as lab tests; Assessment of the patient's problems; and Plan of treatment) was devised to give doctors a reproducible and efficient format to document their thinking and their work.

Unfortunately, this format is not a requirement outside of most training programs, and doctors are often allowed to write whatever they want in their progress notes. A standardized format such as this would make doctors think before they write and would probably improve the level of their patient care.

I didn't realize until much later that "buffing" the charts is as necessary to avoid litigation as it is to provide good care. Many doctors are their own worst enemies because they are careless documenters. They may be excellent doctors, but it really doesn't matter in court unless they can prove it. The "proof is in the charting" rather than in the talking!

We are living in a litigious society where people feel that it is their birthright to sue other people. Sometimes lawsuits are justified and necessary, but at times, suits are initiated out of greed, anger, or a desire to shift responsibility for problems to someone else.

Many people don't want to take responsibility for their actions and want to find someone else to blame for their troubles. We are living in a society that finds little shame in the word "blame."

Attorneys often play more than a small role as instigators by passing out their cards on the doorsteps of hospitals and at accident scenes. It is hard to drive down a freeway, look at a phone book, or watch television without finding ads for personal injury attorneys: "If your baby was born with a birth defect, call your attorney!" Lawyers have helped society equate blame with monetary gain. Hence, blame shifting is commonplace.

Doctors are sometimes perceived as being smug, arrogant, and uncommunicative with their patients. In my experience, most patients can better handle unforeseen outcomes when they feel that the doctor has done his or her best and has taken the time to communicate with them and their loved ones. I want to stress the importance of communication with the family. It takes only **one** upset family member to "upset the apple cart" and initiate a lawsuit.

Unfortunately, doctors are pulled in so many directions and are under so much pressure that they sometimes forget to talk to the patient and sincerely listen to what he or she has to say. Communication is a part of the art of medicine that is difficult to both teach and learn. Not everyone is a good communicator. For some, it is more natural than for others.

It is important for the patient to feel that the doctor has empathy for his or her experiences and that the doctor will take the time to sit and talk. Few doctors realize how appreciated they are for "caring." People will be less likely to sue a person whom they like and if they feel genuinely cared for by that person:

> **"I'd say the most important factor in many of our cases—besides the negligence itself—is the quality of the doctor-patient relationship. People just don't sue doctors they like. In all the years I've been in this business, I've never had a potential client walk in and say, 'I really like this doctor, and I feel terrible about doing it, but I want to sue him.'"[2]**

Proper communication is essential to not only allow doctors to determine what is wrong with their patients but also to proactively prevent lawsuits. A lot of doctors don't realize that communication is the key weapon that they have in their arsenal against attorneys and avoidable lawsuits. It is also what makes them good doctors.

The press has fueled the public's perception that doctors are often not to be trusted. Medicine is a profession where failure is not well tolerated; but what is often seen in the press highlights the worst rather than the best that doctors have to offer. The accidents and mistakes sometimes get more press than the success stories.

People can generally tell if their doctor is a human being who sincerely cares by the way that he talks and acts. Sincerity goes a long way towards calming anger and fear, two common emotions that lead to lawsuits. There is nothing worse than an uncommunicative, uncaring doctor to grease the wheels of jurisprudence.

A doctor needs to attempt to understand his patients' emotions in order to be an effective doctor. This is just common sense and makes for good medical care. It helps both doctor and patient. A corollary to being a better doctor who is liked by his patients is that he will be less likely to be sued in the event of a bad outcome.

Often doctors have a hard time dealing with their own frustrations and anger. They sometimes misdirect their own emotions, usually without malice or forethought towards patients or their families. A lot of doctors are also frustrated by their inability to help their patients adequately due to a healthcare system that is unwieldy and seems to work against them. They also feel the effects of fatigue and pressure and sometimes the stress of their own personal problems.

The weight of the world sometimes transforms itself into frustration and anger, and doctors, being human, are subject to the same problems and emotions as the rest of us. Unfortunately, the doctor's problem is that he can't show his emotions to his patients and at times can't even ventilate to friends and family who really have no way of understanding what he is going through because they "haven't been there."

Unfortunately, there is a small percentage of truly bad doctors out there whose judgment and performance is so poor that it makes the public's general perception of doctors even worse. Some people will do anything for prestige or money, and doctors are surely no exception. But this is a small minority compared to the majority who truly care about their patients and about not ripping off the system.

This small minority abuses the insurance carriers and takes advantage of their patients. These dishonest doctors feed the auditors and the attorneys and make the lives of good and honest doctors miserable. We hear about these doctors more often than we hear about the good ones because they make splashier headlines.

We are living in a technological revolution, and some doctors just haven't kept up with the changes. Patients, by and large, know more about their medical problems than they did a quarter of a century ago. They frequently are prepared with intelligent questions when they visit their doctor, and they demand honest and forthright answers. The doctor-patient relationship needs to be treated as a sacred trust and is so important that it deserves a chapter of its own.

The Internet is a source of information that can allow patients to be more proactive and more informed about their care. Patients now feel empowered and are less shy when it comes to questioning their doctor's performance. A doctor needs to understand the ramifications of this empowerment to stay out of the courtroom and keep pace with his patients.

Doctors can no longer bury themselves in their textbooks and think of themselves as all knowing and above reproach. They need to understand that their patients are consumers who will judge them on the basis of care that they deliver.

Litigation and the common cold have a lot in common: they are both ubiquitous and will find you no matter how hard you try to hide, simply because you are in the wrong place at the wrong time! However, I have learned several important principles over the years that a doctor can follow that may help him to avoid the needless pain and suffering of lawsuits.

Lawyers are often virtually handed lawsuits by the medical profession on silver platters. Taking a blend of vitamin C and Echinacea may help as deterrents for the "common cold" of medical litigation if the following points are remembered:

- Doctors shouldn't try to be heroes. They need to show their patients that they are human if they want credibility. This means admitting that they don't know everything, which happens to be the truth! Patients need to know that their doctor doesn't consider himself to be infallible. Doctors should say, " I don't know the answer to your question, but I will find out and get back to you," rather than faking an answer. When doctors think that they don't need help, they become dangerous. They become even more dangerous when they "cover up" their ignorance with misinformation and even falsehoods.

- Doctors should ask the patient to get a second opinion if they are unsure of a diagnosis or treatment. They should consider asking other doctors for advice if necessary. This is not a sign of weakness but of strength and maturity.
- Communicating on the same level with both the patient and his or her family, preferably by sitting and talking with them face to face, is incredibly important. Both the patients and family can be a doctor's friend or foe in a courtroom. It is just plain good medicine to communicate with both the patient and his or her loved ones. Sometimes families can be challenging and present many obstacles, but more often than not, they facilitate good care.
- Physicians should remember that, above all else, they should "do no harm." Conservative treatment is sometimes the best course. Doctors don't have to offer aggressive or radical treatment, and they should try to put themselves in their patients' shoes when they make their recommendations.
- Doctors often undermine other physicians and healthcare providers by saying things that make themselves look good while making others look bad. I cringe when I hear comments coming from doctors and nurses that are interpreted by the patient or family as being derogatory about a colleague's care. Sometimes these comments are misconstrued by anxious listeners and are not meant to be malicious. Competing physicians in larger cities sometimes say things that give patients the impression that doctors in smaller communities don't provide proper medical care. I have heard horror stories coming from "the big city" filled with negativisms about the quality of care given by other healthcare workers. I have spent countless hours stomping out fires started by other people in my own profession! The true beneficiaries of this kind of talk are

the attorneys. These off-the-cuff comments are potentially disastrous and are litigation inducers. Yes, believe it or not, remarks by doctors and nurses are the leading cause of their own misery in courtrooms.

- Even though being attentive to one's patients sounds overly simplistic, doctors are too often guilty of brushing off their patients' complaints. When patients tell their doctor about their problems, they often indicate when they are upset or angry by not only what they say but also how they say it. An astute listener will pick up on these subtle clues. Patients have even sometimes hinted to me that they are seeking legal advice about another doctor. A resourceful doctor will take this information and deal with problems head on, and proactively, hopefully avoiding future confrontations. It takes a listening ear and a precious commodity called "time." Through careful listening, a doctor can pick up on a variety of emotions from the patient and family, including anger and outright hostility, both of which are common in the victims of serious illness or injury.
- It is important for doctors to avoid venting their own frustrations when dealing with the emotions of the people under their care. The resulting vicious cycle benefits no one and can only hurt the doctor and his relationship with his patients. Doctors need to find other outlets that are not destructive for their frustrations.
- Remember that it is the patient's perception of his or her treatment that matters, not the doctor's. A lot of times, it is the perceived care that gets a doctor into trouble, not just his perceived attitude towards his patients. Arrogance and haughtiness are invitations to the courtroom.
- Overcharging patients is "bad medicine" and gives the profession a "bum rap." It is also playing into the hands

of the press and government who have already stereotyped doctors as moneygrubbers. That is also how lawyers want doctors to be perceived by juries and is a lot more expensive in the long run than adjusting fees or working with patients to help them pay their bills over a period of time. I have a policy in my office to help my patients financially, and I don't charge interest. I let banks do that! However, I have little patience with patients who threaten to sue me if I don't "write off" their charges. I won't allow my patients to use the legal system to coerce or threaten me although some of them would like to use the threat of a lawsuit to get their way.

- Violating the sanctity of the doctor-patient relationship is the kiss of death. It is important to allow patients at all times to maintain their dignity as human beings. Doctors should never deny this basic human need, and they should remember to treat others with the respect that they would themselves desire. There is a basic foundation of trust that needs to be present in the doctor-patient relationship. If this foundation is marred because the doctor disregards his obligations to his patients, he leaves himself open to a myriad of problems, thus destroying his ability to care effectively for his patients. A good rule of thumb is for doctors to remember that they are always their patients' advocates. Being a good doctor means putting your patients' needs and rights first; this will protect him in court and in the examination room.
- Doctors should never hide mistakes or bad results, no matter how tempting it may be to try to find "a way out." This adds to a climate of mistrust and compounds the problem. Patients should never be lied to. This certainly invites legal problems and destroys the trust necessary to maintain a good relationship:

"When a patient has a bad medical result, the doctor has to take the time to explain what happened, and to answer the patient's questions—to treat him like a human being. The doctors who don't are the ones who get sued."[3]

- Physicians should communicate, communicate, and communicate even more! They don't have to be the most knowledgeable or best doctors in the world if this simple advice is followed. It is so important that doctors should consider this to be a basic part of their practice of medicine: a rule to live by.
- It is important for doctors to remember to document in the medical record everything that is said and done in front of patients and their families. The adage is true that "if it was not written, it was not done." Sloppy record keeping is ultimately inferred as malpractice even if a doctor did all the right things in front of his patient. Poor record keeping equals "bad doctor" to most juries and essentially allows doctors to hang themselves. S.O.A.P. notes provide an efficient format and give uniformity to the way doctors express themselves on paper. However, they are not yet required by hospitals and insurance companies. Doctors who already feel over-regulated will probably resist attempts by others to gain further control of what they do.
- Writing legibly sounds incredibly simple and even silly for someone with over twenty years of education. It is something that we all learn in grade school. Yet it is common knowledge that doctors have poor penmanship. Errors and lawsuits are bound to happen if people can't read what is written on the chart. Sloppy handwriting makes doctors appear to be sloppy in the

care of their patients. Why is this the case? I truly think that doctors are so pressured for time that they don't take the time to write and organize their thoughts properly on paper. I now dictate my important notes if I'm in a hurry.

- Doctors need to remember that there are valid reasons for lawsuits, just as there are frivolous ones. They can blame the attorneys only for the latter.
- Lawyers can be a doctor's best friend or worst nightmare. **The choice is a "no-brainer"!**

I have been fortunate to have been sued only once in twenty years although the fear is constantly in the back of my mind. Part of this is luck, but part of the reason is that I take the principles that I have outlined here seriously. Other suits have been threatened, but I have managed to "head them off at the pass" by proactively taking the time to communicate with my patients and their families. This has saved me time and grief in the long run because litigation is very time consuming for a doctor, and costly.

My patient developed a large groin hematoma that unfortunately resulted in nerve injury after a catheterization that I had performed. At his deposition, I discovered that the patient had resented the way that he had been treated. He even disliked the way that I had dressed when I made my rounds, and he felt that I had been arrogant! It was the patient's perception of me that had encouraged the lawsuit. Litigation could possibly have been averted if I had taken the time to communicate better and if I had taken the time to show him that I truly cared about him. He was hurt by what he considered to be a smug attitude on my part, and this perception is what came across in his deposition.

Communication is as much my responsibility as is passing a catheter to clean out a blockage in an artery. I have also learned to try not to be my own worst enemy and to try to avoid giving attorneys any more ammunition than they already have by virtue of their status as lawmakers in our society.

I have learned to treat litigation like the disease that it is: with an ounce of prevention. Lawyers help to spread the disease; they are not the disease itself, nor the enemy.

It is important to spend time with patients; I average about fifteen to twenty minutes per patient in the office as opposed to the five or ten that I hear that other doctors spend with their patients. As a result, my patient-customers don't feel like they are being brushed off. They feel that a genuine interest is being taken in their welfare. I don't do this to avoid litigation; it's just my style. This is the way that I enjoy practicing medicine, even though it is less lucrative. As a by-product of this approach, I feel that I have been sued less frequently than my colleagues.

Recently a patient came to me and told me:

"Dr. Farber, I was going to sue one of your associates, but my attorney told me that I would have to sue you too. I told him No!"

Society needs to take a long look at the senseless and frivolous lawsuits that often clog our courts. These suits can be discouraged by a judicial system that discourages a "nothing to lose" mentality and that limits the size of awards to plaintiffs. Suits can also be discouraged by a careful pre-selection of cases by independent review boards. Clients and attorneys who file frivolous suits that harass others and overburden court dockets need to have a risk of financial loss for their misguided and costly efforts.

When being sued can't be prevented, doctors need to learn to play the "litigation game" as well as their attorney-counterparts. This is difficult because the playing field isn't level. Attorney-politicians generally make up the rules.

A useful strategy is learning to beat lawyers at their own game. At times, this may mean "acting." Lawyers learn how to "act" in front of judges and juries. It's part of their preparation and training. Most doctors are not as good as attorneys at this art because medical school doesn't teach them how to look and sound in front of an audience.

Doctors need to realize that their verbal skills and body language convey an impression that can make or break them in a courtroom or with their patients. If a doctor appears arrogant, smug, or defiant, then he might as well paint a target on his torso for salivating plaintiff's attorneys. Juries are not apt to feel sorry for an arrogant doctor. Nor are they likely to judge him innocent if he can't express his thoughts verbally or on paper.

My goal in a deposition is to give the opposing attorney a vision of a formidable adversary. I want him to think twice about putting me on a witness stand in front of a jury. This means being sincere, honest, confident, and calm. Being calm sometimes takes a lot of acting, but it is important not to let opposing attorneys think they can ruffle your feathers.

If you think that this is not a "high-stakes" game, winner take all, then think again. Lawyers have declared open hunting season against doctors, and it lasts all year!

I dedicate the poem "Right or Wrong" to my attorney-friends who have not only made my life more interesting but have also helped make litigation "The American Way," like Mom and apple pie.

But don't expect to get an extra helping of anything but attorney's fees. If I had only become an attorney before going to medical school, I could have paid myself one heckuva retainer and prevented a lot of headaches over the years!

Right or Wrong?

(Ode to a Litigator)

Are you friend or foe?
I really don't know.
When you wrong a right,
Can you sleep at night?
Right or wrong, wrong or right
Can you sleep all right?

Charge by the minute
There's no sin in it.
After all, it's all right to
Right a wrong, or is it,
Wrong a right?
Can you sleep all night?
Or just by the minute,
After all,
There's no sin in it.

"To Err Is Human?"

Doctors and nurses are human, just like the rest of us. But unfortunately, the mistakes made by the medical profession are a lot more glaring to the public, and we are less tolerant of them when we compare them to the mistakes of others. Iatrogenic problems are created by the medical profession and cause a patient to get even sicker as a result of usually well-intentioned treatment. It is extremely frustrating for me to hear that someone has been the victim of a problem that wouldn't have occurred if the doctor hadn't interfered in the first place. Let me give you a brief example.

Tom was admitted to the hospital with pneumonia. As a result of the treatment with antibiotics, he developed a severe super-infection of his bowel called pseudomembraneous colitis. This required further antibiotics and a central line. The central-line stick caused a pneumothorax, which required a chest tube to be inserted to expand the lung. That chest tube site then became infected, so on, and so forth....

This patient is an unfortunate victim of our technology. Sometimes to cure one problem, we cause others along the way. The question is: How many of these are preventable?

Years of experience have allowed me to see how easily mistakes can happen, even to the best of us. Mistakes are not the same as negligence. Negligence is defined in *Webster's New World College Dictionary* as "a habitual failure to do the right thing, or a carelessness in manner or appearance; indifference."[4] The legal definition is slightly different but implies damage or injury resulting when a reasonable amount of care is not provided.

Part of my former job as the Chairman of Cardiology in my hospital is to investigate these situations and try to find answers and solutions to help prevent future mistakes and complications. Unfortunately, I have concluded that bad things happen to good people, including both good patients and good doctors.

But there are also preventable errors, such as giving the wrong medications or the wrong dosages, things that can be eliminated by further education and by increasing self-awareness. Reducing fatigue and stress can also prevent these errors. I haven't met any doctors or nurses who want to be negligent or who intentionally want to make mistakes. But these unfortunate errors usually happen for a reason.

A report recently published by the Institute of Medicine (IOM) states that errors cause between 44,000 and 98,000 deaths every year in American hospitals![5] This report has rightfully prompted a demand for accountability and an investigation into how these errors might be prevented. Superficially this sounds like a great idea! But wait. It's not that simple.

Hospitals and insurance companies are launching initiatives to prevent errors. Most physicians are not complacent about this topic, as some might suggest. Peer review is in place in most hospitals in order to help with this problem. However, there are some problems that need to be addressed before a dramatic reduction in medical errors can occur.

The IOM report recommends the "confidential, voluntary reporting of injuries due to medical care." This is similar to an approach used by the National Aeronautics and Space Administration for near misses in flight. It also supports some degree of federally mandated public disclosure of serious errors. The criteria for this public reporting are vague.

I can understand the need for the public to know about serious medical mistakes as this knowledge might influence decisions about the public's care. Why is this knowledge or disclosure dangerous to the medical profession? The answers are simple and logical once you have a basic understanding of the American legal system.

How many doctors would honestly want to disclose their own errors, or the errors of others, knowing the potential ramification this could have on their own careers and futures? Lawyers are waiting in the darkness of night, ready to pounce on the perpetrators of even honest errors. There needs to be a leash on lawsuits.

The sincere and honest reporting of errors serves no purpose unless the results are used to help reduce the incidence of future events. Believe me, I'm all in favor of that! However, this reporting will be incomplete and will never scratch the surface of the problem until doctors feel free to report these errors without the fear of retribution that takes the form of malpractice litigation.

This does not give doctors an excuse for dishonesty. Quite the contrary; doctors need to address the issue of medical errors, and especially negligence, with vigor, openness, and a sense of purpose and not leave it to the legal profession. Why? The answer is easy: it is the right thing to do.

Doctors and hospitals need to find methods of prevention that are cost effective and affordable. They need to hold themselves accountable for their errors because lawyers will be more than happy to do the job for them. But who will pay for these changes and new safety measures? Will the government or the insurance companies pay for the systems that will have to be put in place to prevent complications and medical errors?

Current fiscal constraints will make it difficult for any entity to absorb these costs.

> **"Preventing adverse events will be a matter of creativity, commitment, and dollars. Nurses and doctors can provide the creativity and commitment, but the dollars, especially for computerized prevention systems, are increasingly scarce."[6]**

Tort reform is a prerequisite for providing better health care. Hopefully, both the medical profession and the government will address the funding of programs to determine the best ways of making healthcare professionals less vulnerable to committing human errors.

Revamping our system of medical education and improving staffing in hospitals may reduce the errors caused by fatigue and exhaustion. Overworked doctors and nurses are certainly more vulnerable to making mistakes that can be prevented. We need to reduce the pressures of our current system that shortchanges our manpower and stretches people to, and often beyond, their limits of endurance. Stress plus fatigue is commonplace in medicine, and is a time bomb waiting to go off!

Let's not forget that we are all human. Doctors and nurses are no different than anyone else in that regard. Remember that doctors, like Superman, have their kryptonite. Fatigue and an overdose of ego can be a dangerous combination.

But as a society, we must also put an end to the witch-hunts!

How "She Got the Gold Mine and I Got the Shaft"

> **"It is often stated that marriage is work and we are warned that the three most common marital problems are about sex, money, and in-laws. Most of us underestimate the amount of tenacity involved in living and compromising with another human being on a daily basis. Physicians and their spouses, in addition to the problems common in all marriages, face unique problems related to their personalities and profession..."[7]**

Don't become a statistic!

Medicine is truly a jealous mistress. She doesn't like it when too much time is spent away from her. The old axiom is true that "you can't live with her, and you can't live without her." She provides a challenge to any relationship that competes with her needs, and her needs can be too overwhelming at times! She can be a very possessive and destructive mistress if you allow her to rule your life. I learned this the hard way.

You would think that someone who had gone through twenty-five years of education would be a quick learner. Wrong! It's amazing that someone can be so successful in one aspect of his life and be such a slow learner in areas that involve "living." I have asked myself over and over again how I could be such a good doctor and still have a personal life that could be considered self-induced purgatory. I didn't particularly like the answers.

I have been divorced four times, so I can claim to be somewhat of a layman's expert on the subject. I am not bragging about the fact that I should have written the song, "She Got the Gold Mine; I Got the Shaft," because I have sung it over and over again.

I hope that I can shed a little light from my own experiences about divorce in the medical profession and about how our legal system treats divorce and those who are suffering through it. More importantly, I would like to discuss how doctors and their spouses might cope with their lives so that divorce might become less commonplace and so that you won't wind up like me...a victim of the legal profession and a casualty of divorce.

After reading the first few chapters of this book, it is probably not hard to see why doctors and divorce are frequent companions. A medical career ultimately tests most marriages, and many newlyweds are totally unaware of the challenges they are about to face.

When a person marries a doctor, she marries someone who dedicates the majority of his waking hours to being around other people: she marries into a demanding profession. At times, it seems as if everything and everybody else comes in second place to the advancement of the doctor's career. Sometimes this causes resentment on the part of the non-doctor spouse.

Marriage requires a lot of patience, perseverance, self-esteem, and understanding. Medical marriages, in particular, are not meant for the fainthearted or for those who want their spouses home at exactly 5 P.M. for dinner. It's important for doctors and their spouses to understand their own needs as well as their partner's and realize what they are getting into before they take the leap.

Love often blinds people to reality, and it makes all of us wear rose-colored glasses at one time or another. The truth is that medical marriages are inherently difficult. It is imperative to understand your own insecurities and jealousies as well as the expectations that you have of your marriage and your partner.

It is important to have good self-esteem for any marriage to work. In the case of a medical marriage, your identity melds into being a doctor's wife or husband. Bev Meninger describes the spouse's position as "living on the edge of the spotlight."[8] Some can adjust to this role, and some simply cannot. It takes a strong sense of "who you are" and good self-esteem to accept the role of a doctor's spouse. Conversations with friends and acquaintances sometimes go like this:

"So you are the doctor's wife. You really don't need to work, do you? How nice; I know you must love being married to such a respected and hard-working man!"

It helps to be able to say, "My life and my happiness don't depend on how late you work tonight." Jealousy tends to be magnified when your spouse has to run back to the hospital in the middle of the night or repeatedly gets home at odd hours. Experience has taught me that there are things that can be done to ease a spouse's insecurities, things that I previously took for granted and that can build trust.

I have also learned not to build false hopes and make promises that I can't keep, such as, "Honey, I promise to be home for dinner." That usually turns into, "Sorry, Dear, another emergency came up from out of nowhere," or possibly even no phone call at all if an emergency occurs.

"I'll try to be home early enough to tuck the kids into bed" may turn into a rare event. Even the most understanding spouses have limits to their endurance and understanding. Sometimes "love just isn't enough," at least not by itself.

For those of you who are curious (and I know you are out there), I take a lot of the blame for my divorces. I did things that I am not proud of, which resulted in a lot of human grief and hurt. I selfishly felt that my work came first and that everyone else needed to sacrifice for my career. I was too naïve and immature to understand my own needs and insecurities.

My hours were long, and they grew even longer when I was unhappy because I received more positive reinforcement from being a doctor than from an unhappy home. The result was a vicious, predictable cycle where there were no winners and only losers, myself included.

I also was attracted to women with whom I shared my long hours. Some of them were nurses who "seemed" to understand what I did and how I felt better than anyone; I want to stress the word **seemed** because people can seem to be a lot of things that they are not. The plain truth is that it is easy for doctors to spend more time working with the medical staff than they spend with their spouses. This is an open door to jealousy and temptation, both of which will destroy a relationship.

There are people of both sexes who put their own self-interests and gain ahead of everything and everyone else. Sometimes they are referred to as "barracudas" and "sharks." I am convinced that they have a unique radar detector for anyone with an "M.D." after their name. They love the money and the prestige that go along with the title of being a doctor's spouse.

Getting dates suddenly became easy once I became a medical student and even easier once I became a doctor. There was suddenly no shortage of people to spend my time with, but the problem was that my ego couldn't handle it. Social success was something that hadn't come easily to me in high school and college when I had been rather introverted and shy. The result was that I wasn't very selective in my decision-making. And yes, I was looking for nurturing to ease the pain of my own psyche.

The truth, though, is that a person is vulnerable to temptation only if he or she is open to it on a conscious or subconscious level. You have to swim in treacherous waters before a shark can bite you. Navigating carefully and avoiding predators is the best way to avoid the catastrophe of being bitten.

My parents raised me to be a trusting but very naïve soul. The result is that I tended to believe the things that I wanted to believe in my relationships with others. I had selective hearing and vision and filtered out the things that my brain didn't want to hear and see. The trusting side of my nature has been both my ally and my enemy, leading me down the primrose path in marriage several times. However, I am convinced that "trust" has made me a better doctor because I share this side of my nature with my patients.

The reasons behind the marriages are as complex as the reasons for their failures. Behind all four marriages was a common thread: I needed to be with someone to feel good about myself. I was "**unhappy with** me." There was obviously something that had to be fixed inside of me before I could be happy in marriage or, for that matter, in any relationship. Unfortunately, I didn't understand this until after numerous trips around the block and after multiple rounds of counseling.

Being married was a way of sharing the trials and tribulations of my life with another human being. Fatigue increased my insecurities and made my important decisions even more difficult. The bottom line was that I was looking for someone who would make me feel better about myself. But it never happened because it was an impossible mission.

I am hoping that someone reading this may learn from my mistakes. Temptation goes with the territory of being a doctor and is hard to ignore. It is also important to be able to spot the barracudas and sharks; they are usually in disguise!

Unfortunately, my trusting nature allowed me to fall into traps that could have been avoided. After years of being a doctor, I have realized that medicine exploits not only a person's strengths but also his or her weaknesses. Being a doctor allows a person to be vulnerable to his or her insecurities because of the stresses and temptations that go with the territory.

My divorces left me in emotional and financial ruin as well as physically and mentally drained. It is hard enough to be a doctor without the additional stress of divorce, but medicine became the escape valve for my unhappiness, allowing me to think of things other than my personal problems.

It allowed me to become, in a real sense, numb to reality. When things got rough at home, I just slipped away into another world, a world where I felt like I was in control and was king.

My second divorce gave attorneys their dream case. I was a young doctor with a good income who had made mistakes in judgment. I was a wonderful target for attorneys and, in the case of a particularly nasty divorce, a wife who was hell-bent on revenge and securing her future.

The divorce became one of the worst nightmares that I have ever had to endure. My white coat had opened the door to a living hell; it was inviting predators instead of offering protection.

Since the attorneys had money to work with, I was forced to endure private investigators and endless hours in deposition. To make matters worse, I was exposed to public ridicule in an open courtroom. Fortunately, many of the accusations against me were unfounded and untrue.

But the innuendos, lies, and accusations caused damage to my reputation that took years to mend, and I felt that I had hit rock bottom. My self-image sank to even lower depths because I felt shame and humiliation. The emotional price of all this was staggering!

The legal system has particularly harsh penalties for doctors and others who are in upper income brackets. Divorces that could easily be over within a few months often drag out for years, usually lasting until every dollar is drained from the till. There are no winners, only losers. I felt emotionally and financially raped, violated, and exploited. To this day, I don't believe that it benefited any one other than the gods of jurisprudence.

A lot of people pass judgment on you when you are a doctor who is divorced. This is especially true in a small community where gossip and rumors are prevalent. It doesn't help to have divorce be a matter of public record, but in our society, very little is private. Many of us believe what we hear. Accusations are often equated with the truth.

To this day, my friends don't hesitate to remind me how many times I have been divorced. This is usually in the weak disguise of a joke. Unfortunately, it was difficult at first to let things "roll off my back," and I took the comments personally for years.

I have learned to laugh off the sarcastic quips and separate them from the good-natured teasing from my friends. My friends usually don't hesitate to tell me when they have heard my other song on the radio: "All My Exes Live in Texas."

But the good news is that we can exorcise our demons! The answers were not easily found and came from both hard work and painful experiences. Finding happiness "from within" instead of "from without" can be very difficult. It takes an honest realization that something has to be done to end the vicious cycle of pain and suffering for everyone involved.

Medical marriages are inherently difficult, and, unfortunately, doctors have a high rate of relationship failure and divorce. The issues in my life reflect many of the issues that people in the medical profession face, but the problems with marriage are complex and identifiable. Let me touch upon the main problems, some of which I have already described.

First, there is the problem of time away from one's family. Doctors spend long hours with co-workers, many of them of the opposite sex. Solace from members of the opposite sex is not hard to find as a crutch if you're looking for it.

It is also "easy" to stay away from an unhappy home and from spending the time necessary to make a marriage work. Doctors spend more time tending to sick patients than to their own sick relationships. They put their own emotional and physical health last.

There is also the issue of what I feel is a common underlying medical personality that tends to put work first and everything else "on the back burner." It is easy to say that problems at home will be worked out later when there is enough time. That time often never comes unless you make it a **priority** and not leave it to chance.

Speaking from experience, it is easy to leave a spouse with more than his or her fair share of responsibility for keeping the home fires burning. Some doctors, unfortunately, are full-time caregivers at work and absentee caregivers at home. Priorities seem to get reversed easily.

Precious little time is spent at home during medical training and while building a practice. Building a marriage comes in second to establishing a career. Non-physician spouses can only carry the burden for the marriage for so long. Intimacy takes a back seat to the daily struggle just to cope and survive the stress and fatigue.

Then there are the pervasive problems of depression, anxiety, and burnout that victimize those in the medical profession. These can spell trouble for a marriage that is already hanging by a thread.

Instead of a synergistic marriage, there is synergistic stress, and this can be disastrous. One plus one suddenly equals less than two. No marriage can survive this equation for too long.

Marriage has to be a blend of independence and interdependence, with the right amount of each. It is hard to have a "working" relationship when the co-workers are burned out from stress and frustration.

Unfortunately, doctors often compound the stresses by not getting the help they need to deal with their own problems. They are too busy surviving the ordeal of residency or medical practice to take time out to seek counseling. Financial problems and constraints for those in training make it difficult for many couples to get the help that is necessary for their relationships.

It is also common to be in denial and think that things will just work out in time. Delayed gratification becomes the order of the day. "Things will get better later when more money comes in and when we have more time together."

Doctors are often workaholics who find it easy to bury their heads in the sand and then rationalize their actions by saying that they are helping mankind and striving for excellence. It is also easier to pass the blame onto others rather than take personal responsibility for important problems and issues.

As I have pointed out in the first three chapters, it is easy to hide behind the disguise of the white coat and not look in the mirror at the person underneath it. Personal renewal is important both for doctors and for their families. Stephen Covey's *The 7 Habits of Highly Effective Families*[9] should be required reading in medical school. It is far more practical and applicable to life than most courses that doctors are required to take as prerequisites. And the principles are definitely not "rocket science."

Let me stress several important lessons that I have learned from years of divorce and remarriage (and tons of experience with attorneys and ex-wives):

- It is crucial for doctors to understand their own emotional and physical needs as well as the needs of their spouse and family. They also must understand their expectations from marriage. Both the doctor and spouse need to be realistic about the inherent difficulties of a medical marriage and deal honestly and openly with them at the very beginning.
- It is important to keep priorities between work and home life in the right order and realize that work is a

"means to an end" and not an end in itself. It definitely is not a substitute for a home life or "having a life." Work is necessary to provide clothing, shelter, and food, but it doesn't improve family relationships. Money definitely does not buy happiness.

- It is critical to budget time. The bottom line is that your kids and spouse need you more than your patients! Doctors all have tremendous demands on their time. It is one of our most precious commodities as human beings, and it is in limited supply. It is important to spend it wisely, not foolishly. One of the most common complaints of medical marriages is a lack of time together.
- Every person needs to take care of his own health before he can tend to that of his family. This means that we need to empower ourselves to take charge of our physical, emotional, and spiritual needs. Renewal is needed in all these areas and is necessary for growth and happiness.
- It is important to resist the temptations that come with the territory of a profession that takes you away from your family for long periods of time. Learning to recognize these temptations and dealing with them accordingly is crucial to a medical marriage.
- Doctors are often socially naïve. Their social skills are often lacking in both dating relationships and marriage. This leads to mistakes in judgment, such as picking the wrong partner and "looking for love in all the wrong places." The rose-colored glasses need to be removed once in a while.
- Doctors should consider getting prenuptial agreements and incorporating their businesses, even if they are convinced that their marriages will be solid. We all like to think positively but being realistic is important. I found myself singing "She Got the Gold Mine; I Got

the Shaft" because I let my heart overrule my head, and I didn't follow the advice of friends and attorneys who tried to convince me to protect my assets. No matter how much faith you have in people, there are, unfortunately, people who will marry a doctor because he or she is a doctor and divorce a doctor because he or she is a doctor. There are plenty of attorneys out there who will be paid a handsome price to help them.

- We should always remember that the only ones who profit from divorce are the attorneys; everyone else suffers emotionally, physically, spiritually, and economically. Whole families, including children, are left devastated and irreparably harmed.
- Remember that the effects of the divorce will remain forever, both from an emotional and economic standpoint. Then decide if it is really worth it or if it would be better to work hard to make your marriage work.
- It is important to remember that the non-doctor spouse or significant other has an identity. Help him or her to recognize his or her potential and try to understand that his or her happiness will lead to your happiness as well. Don't expect your partner or your family to sacrifice forever.

It took four divorces to force me to look at the person behind my white coat, to acknowledge that he has weaknesses as well as strengths. I really had no choice after I hit rock bottom and realized that I was sinking. Subsequent to my divorces, I was forced to file bankruptcy and was close to both financial and emotional ruin. Abraham Lincoln's sentiments reflected my own experiences when he proclaimed:

"I have been driven many times to my knees by the overwhelming conviction that I had nowhere else to go."

Fortunately, hard work, prayer, and "father time" have healed the wounds of divorce, but some effects linger and will never disappear. There are scars and terrible memories of days in court that I pray will stop torturing me; these reminders have haunted me in nightmares. My medical practice has survived, but more importantly, I have found loyal patients and friends who have stuck with me despite my personal trials and tribulations.

Divorce can also be very enlightening when it comes to testing friendships and loyalty in relationships. You learn to differentiate the trusting friends from those who are superficial acquaintances. It helps to remember that "real friends are those who, when you've made a fool of yourself, don't feel that you've done a permanent job." Multiply that times four, and you will find that your best and truest friends are the ones that stick by you...repeatedly.

Ironically, divorce can teach us painful lessons about love, and it can also teach us about life's second chances. My family and children have stuck by me and shown me what love is all about. Most importantly, I had to learn to love myself and be willing to give myself a second chance.

Before I could put my divorce behind me, I needed to also learn to laugh at myself and be able to find humor in my own failures and mistakes. Humor is therapeutic and heals a lot of emotional and physical wounds. I have had to learn to forgive myself, and I have also needed to "exorcise my exes" before I could go on with my life: "We play God when we do not forgive ourselves or others."

Before I finish this section, I want to say a few words about attorneys. I am sure that many of you think that I dislike attorneys and that what you are reading is a reflection of my bad experiences with the legal profession and my desire to taste the sweetness of revenge. Wrong!

There are both honest and dishonest doctors and attorneys. Both professions are in a position to do much harm and much good by their actions. Both can cause whole families to be devastated through loss and emotional distress. Doctors and lawyers can both succumb to conflicts of interest.

I hope that the future will allow a system that is based on agreement rather than dispute. My experiences with our current system of "injustice" have shown me that we are not very close to that goal. Right now, there is too much financial gain to be made by provoking dispute rather than seeking alternatives, one of which is called "mediation." Mediation is a highly successful method of promoting agreement and compromise, but it is underutilized because lawyers don't profit from it as much as from the traditional approach.

There should be a flat fee for divorces, not an hourly wage that causes families to remain in divorce court for years while attorneys' pockets are padded. Doctors' fees are dictated by both the federal and state government (Medicare and Medicaid) as well as by the insurance industry, which pays them what they think their work is worth. They are paid the same for an operation or procedure irrespective of its level of difficulty. Should attorneys be held to a lesser standard of accountability, especially when their fees can devastate families just like an illness? Should the rich in our society be able to obtain better legal protection or medical care than the poor?

There should be time limitations on divorce, not only for financial but also for emotional reasons. People have to be allowed to bring closure to emotionally distressing issues.

Our current system makes this very difficult. Most of my divorced physician friends have had divorce marathons that lasted for years. This is disastrous to the lives of everyone involved, especially the children because Mom and Dad can't go on with their lives, and therefore they can't either. Children are the innocent victims of divorce and are often caught in the middle and used as pawns by attorneys and vengeful spouses.

Divorce becomes an endurance contest, a test of who's going to blink first. I traded money to get on with my life. It was an expensive tradeoff, but after two years of living with fear and chaos, it was a necessity for my spiritual and mental health. Of course, lawyers have all the time in the world. (That's especially true if you are paid an hourly wage!)

"Dirty" tactics by attorneys should be punished. Judges' decisions may be easily swayed by what is politically expedient. A system that allows so much personal carnage and ruin needs to change.

By the way, some of my family and best friends are attorneys. My sister is a judge, and I love her dearly despite her profession. Lawyers have helped me far more than they have hurt me over the past twenty years. I have decided that I like them better as my friends than as my worst enemies and nightmares.

All I know is that when I am seeking to right a wrong, I go to the best darn attorney I can find. Sometimes in life, defining the hero and the villain depends on your perspective.

I hope that you don't find yourself singing one of my songs at the end of the day. It's wonderful therapy but can get pretty monotonous if you sing it too often. While you're at it, don't forget to like yourself, forgive yourself, and laugh at yourself along the way.

I have dedicated a rather special poem to a few of my exes:

My Vexing Exes

Exes can come in both sexes.
My ex-files total exactly four;
Lord—I don't need anymore
To sharpen and grind their axes!

Extraordinary expectations from these exes
I find not exhilarating or extremely funny.
As my exes extract a lot of support and alimony,
And give me ulcers for which I take prilosecs.

Sing my song and laugh if you will.
All my exes do live in Texas.
I have even exorcised them with hexes,
But they exhaust and perplex me still.

"A Fool and His Money...."

The next gator is a sly, slick, and sometimes sleazy fellow. You might talk to him on the phone and not even know what he looks like. He comes in many disguises, sometimes hiding under cover by day and spending your money with the ease of dialing a cell phone.

He looks for your weak spots, and he takes advantage of the fact that doctors are so busy that they let others spend their money for them. He might even be your distant cousin or a long-lost friend. He may dress like a businessman or an attorney. The disguises are limitless, but his main goal is to separate a fool from his money.

Like a lot of doctors, I didn't take any business courses in high school or college. They didn't offer any in medical school. I was too busy studying anatomy and physiology and reading Shakespeare to even realize the importance that business and economics would have in my career or in planning my future.

I took all the courses that were required to get into med school, but few of them dealt with practical matters relating to survival. I had no idea that being a good doctor was one thing and that being a doctor who was a good businessman was something quite different.

Youthfulness didn't give me the foresight to understand that it takes financial know-how to survive in this world. It wasn't until later that I discovered that life's not just about being good at what you do.

Understanding finance is as essential a skill in the real world as is learning a career. When I was a college student, I was too concerned with the war in Vietnam and with getting into medical school to care about the stock market, how to run a business, or plan for retirement.

As a result, I left school well read and knowledgeable about how to be a doctor but totally naïve about something very important called "money." That "green stuff" wasn't the reason why I was becoming a doctor anyway. My goal was to go out in the world and help people; my youthful idealism steered me away from the boring world of finance. I was young, and retirement was years away. Nothing to worry about!

Soon after I graduated, people approached me with "get-rich-quick schemes." They talked circles around me, and I only half understood what they meant. They sounded good, and I believed many of them. As a result, I made more financial mistakes than I care to admit. I was a sucker for the proverbial sales pitch. I was naïve, a babe in the woods, and was not at all street-smart. I trusted in others to lead me to the pot of treasure at the end of the rainbow.

My financial fiascos included an oil deal, proposed by my accountant, that turned out later to consist of dry and fake wells. I was involved in litigation for three years as a result of this scam. My cousin encouraged me to become a partner in an apartment complex that eventually went bankrupt when the oil economy went sour. The experience taught me a valuable lesson about doing business with my relatives; business and family sometimes don't mix.

A broker in New York got me to invest over the telephone in stock options. Right!! You guessed it! I lost all my money as a result of talking to a man that I have never met to this day!

I receive phone calls regularly from investors and brokers who want to earn a commission by helping me invest my money "wisely." I didn't know how to say the word "no!" My youthful idealism made me want to believe in people. Often my trust was misplaced.

All of these errors culminated in a bankruptcy that was embarrassing and ego bruising. I wondered how a successful doctor, after twenty years of medical practice, could find himself being rejected when applying for a simple credit card. How could I be refused credit when I was considered successful by most standards set by society?

There were several reasons for this. I spent way too much money on frivolous things that I thought I should have to keep up my image, such as a Jaguar and a BMW. My financial woes were compounded by divorces that took away half of my medical practice and a large portion in legal fees and alimony payments.

In the early years of my medical practice, I was "**a kid in a candy store**." I had never seen so much money before, and I didn't know what to do with it when I finally found out how to make it. Money burned a hole in my pocket and literally fell out (or into other people's hands!).

I have loaned money to friends, never to see a trace of it again, and I never stopped to think that I needed to protect myself in the event that the debtor would skip town or file for bankruptcy.

Sometimes there is a fine line between ignorance and stupidity. I certainly didn't use much "horse sense" in my financial dealings. I made myself into a very friendly bank that gave out unsecured loans at low interest rates. If I had been a bank, I would have gone out of business in a hurry! Declaring bankruptcy is no fun. It was, and always will be, one of the lowest points of my life.

To be fair, you need to know more about my background. I will reiterate what it is like to be a doctor. I am not asking for your sympathy because a lot of people work very hard just making it from day to day in life, scratching and clawing for everything they get.

Doctors make more money than most people. However, as you can see from my earlier chapters, becoming a doctor takes years of hard work. And like many other professions, being a doctor requires putting in long hours, depending on your specialty and nature of your practice.

Dinners and families are frequently left alone at the table; warm beds become cold in the middle of the night. The days of telling patients to "take two aspirin and call in the morning" are over (if they ever really existed), although aspirin is one of the first things that is given to heart attack victims!

Lengthy and grueling years of training often are transformed into long hours managing a busy medical practice and taking care of patients. Both are full-time jobs and can keep one working twelve to fourteen hours a day and taking call for weeks at a time without a break.

At times, it is a twenty-four-hour-a-day profession, and there is little time for anything else. Work follows me wherever I go. My family and I are often like two ships passing in the night. In spite of this, and after almost twenty years of medical practice, I am still far from financial independence. And I have no one else to blame but myself.

Although doctors are higher on the ladder of financial success when compared to most, they are not even close to those in other walks of life in terms of an hourly wage. This is especially true in the new world of managed care and Medicare.

Overheads have skyrocketed as a result of increasing malpractice premiums. Increased staffing is required to deal with the mountainous volumes of paper work that have resulted from the need to comply with the regulations of managed-care companies and governmental agencies. Doctors generally consume more working hours to make the same income that they made ten years ago.

You see, I did what I was taught to do, which was to succeed at becoming a compassionate and caring doctor. That was my number-one priority throughout a good part of my life. My training and intuition never led me towards anything else.

I was taught how to pass tests, not how to "pass life." Business courses were never required, and my ivory-tower training insulated me well from the reality that most people experienced at much younger ages.

"Never having enough time" has been an almost insurmountable problem. There is only so much time in a given day, and quite a bit of it is spent doing what I love and worked hard to do.

Securing my family's future is a much higher priority now than in the past. I enjoy investing, and I enjoy reading *The Wall Street Journal.* Like that song says: "If I only knew then what I didn't know now."

I no longer take calls from brokers and advisors that I have never met. I now research my investments as thoroughly as possible. Learning about the world of finance has actually been challenging and fun! It takes me away from thinking about sickness and illness and is an important outlet for my psyche.

I have learned to protect my ASSets. Asset protection is critical for doctors and should be taught as part of a medical curriculum, along with basic business management and financial planning.

Experience has taught me that ignorance is definitely not bliss. I learned the hard way that I could still put trust in others while not burying my head in the sand. Blind trust can be dangerous to your health. I have learned to protect myself from those who would abuse it.

As W.C. Fields so aptly put it: "**Trust everybody, but cut the cards.**"

I am approached almost daily by charities that need and deserve my help. I owe a good part of my living to people who are less fortunate. God put me in this world to help people in anyway that I can: medically, spiritually, and financially. That doesn't mean, though, that I should allow them to help themselves.

I have come to the conclusion that a lot of people feel they are entitled to others' bank accounts. Is there a big bull's-eye painted on doctors' foreheads (or their backs)? Sometimes, I feel like I am being used for target practice!

The irony is that now, managed care and the government have staked a claim on a lot of the money that doctors used to make before it even gets into their pockets!

Through all of my experiences, I remain somewhat idealistic and believe that helping people has a special reward that can't be measured in dollars and cents.

However, idealism only goes so far when you are paying the bills. Watch out for moochers and bloodsuckers! Doctors still have their leeches.

A "Simple" Case of Embezzlement

This gray-haired, wrinkled woman was like a mother to me. I was a busy doctor, and my sixty-five-year-old office manager had my full trust. She helped me to keep my practice together by working late balancing the books, paying the bills, depositing money into my bank account, and making sure that billing was done accurately. I was certain that my accountant was watching over what she was doing, and I really was not very concerned when things were "tight." She was also my friend and my confidant. We had made it through tough times before.

I felt secure with the notion that my medical practice was in good hands while I worked long hours doing what I did and liked best, being a doctor. I didn't particularly care for the business end of the practice anyway, so it was easy to let her run with the ball when it came to all this other mundane stuff.

My accountant approached me with what later turned out to be one of the most painful discoveries of my life. My surrogate mother-office manager had not only used my credit card to buy a cruise for her family, but she had used it as well to purchase numerous other personal items for herself and for her family. The bills were then paid out of my corporate account with checks that I never saw. I was stunned and refused to believe what my ears had heard. Not a woman that I had complete faith in and had come to love!

It turned out to be a cold, calculated, and blood-chilling deception. I had buried my head in the sand while a person whom I had completely trusted had robbed me blind. I hadn't safeguarded my business interests from embezzlement. I was too busy being a doctor to tend to the daily necessities of running a business.

It has taken me years to recover my financial losses, and the litigation probably will last until I am old and gray. A by-product of this experience is that I now sign my own checks and watch over the books myself. It was a hard lesson to learn about both life and trust.

This experience rocked the foundation of my life more than my four divorces and bankruptcy. How could I have been so wrong in placing so much faith in another person? It made me question my own judgment and put to the test my faith in God and in human nature.

It has been one of the saddest experiences of my life. But I learned from it and went on with my life, hopefully a bit wiser.

Managed Care: Are We Trying to Buy a Cadillac for the Price of a Motor Scooter?

Just when I thought that I had learned how to cope with disease and suffering, I was introduced to something even more complex and disturbing: managed care. Its many faces and names sound like something that only a science-fiction writer could invent.

The initials are confusing, even for the most erudite among us. Few doctors and patients really understand how it works. It is like a virus that plagues the medical profession and, arguably, society as a whole. It frustrates and baffles me as much as, or more than, the diseases that I have been trained to treat. I now realize that all those years of schooling never prepared me for anything as complex or enigmatic as the subject that I am about to discuss.

I chuckle to myself when I hear people hint that doctors go into medicine for "the money." I won't argue that most doctors have a high standard of living; however, most don't have the vast fortunes or endless resources that some people associate with the medical profession because of its past reputation. Managed care and the government have changed all that. And so have doctors themselves!

What is the purpose of managed care? Managed care was born in an attempt to cut the spiraling costs of health care and to try to make doctors and hospitals accountable for what they do and make them responsible to "an unprejudiced third party."

These ideas are noble but have had numerous effects that are also quite negative on both patients and the doctors who care for them. The actual result has also been that patient care has been taken out of the hands of doctors and put into the hands of big business.

Doctors can blame themselves for a lot of the managed-care problem. For years, they ordered tests and used technology without any financial accountability. But there are a lot of other reasons behind the tremendous healthcare costs that we experience.

Both the legal and medical professions need to take partial responsibility for the fix that we are in. I'll tell you more about the "hidden costs" of health care in a minute, but first let me give you a little more background about the complexities of managed care.

Learning about managed care is a veritable sea of alphabet soup. There are all kinds of initials for people to become familiar with. Terms such as **HMO's**, **PPO's**, **PCP's**, and **IPA's** are examples of everyday jargon and sources of confusion for doctors and their patients alike.

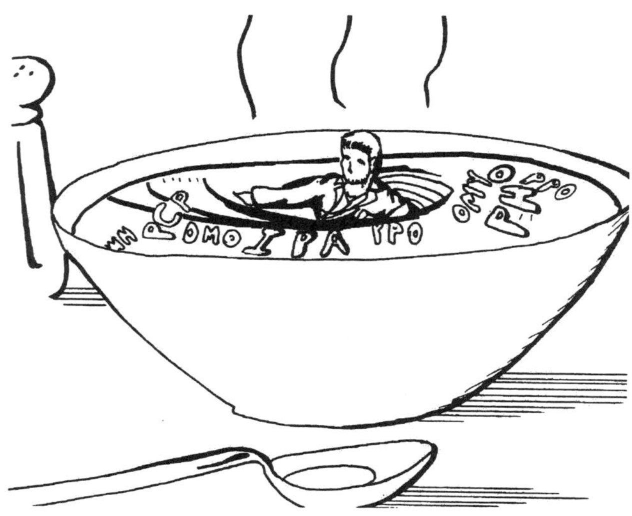

An HMO is a **Health Maintenance Organization** that is essentially a product line sold by insurance companies to employers and individuals. To make matters even more complicated, there are several types of HMO's available.

They are the following: Commercial HMO's, whose members are of working age and employed; Medicare HMO's whose members have elected to not participate in the government-sponsored Medicare program and have assigned their Medicare benefits to a licensed HMO; and finally, Medicaid HMO's whose members qualify to receive government-supported benefits through Medicaid but are mandated to receive services through a licensed HMO.

HMO's generally offer the lowest premiums available, except for the Medicare and Medicaid HMO's whose premiums are paid by the government. They also offer the most limited networks of providers. Providers are hospitals, physicians, and ancillary personnel who have contracted with HMO's at a discounted rate in exchange for patient direction and volume. These providers who are contracted are referred to as a network. The members of the network are limited in number to aid in controlling costs.

The insured patient is required to select a PCP, or primary care provider, whose name is provided as being in the network. PCP's are generally physicians who practice family medicine, internal medicine, pediatrics, or, in some cases, obstetrics and gynecology.

PCP's are the coordinators of patient care, giving referrals when indicated to specialists and facility providers who also participate in the network. PCP's are generally referred to as "gatekeepers."

PCP's are contracted by most HMO's to work on a "capitated" basis. Under the terms of a capitated contract, the PCP will receive a per-member-per-month (PMPM) payment by the HMO for each member assigned to that PCP.

For example, if a PCP has 150 members assigned to him/her at a payment of $10 per patient, then the PCP will receive a check each month in the amount of $1,500. The PCP will receive this $1,500 per month no matter how many of the 150 patients are seen or how much work is done on them. The PCP assumes "financial risk" for these patients. Some specialists are also capitated by some HMO's. Generally, no benefits are paid if patients go "out of network" and see doctors who are not in the plan.

In some instances, IPA's, or independent practice associations, contract with physician providers. In an IPA scenario, the IPA contracts with the insurance company, and the IPA, as a medical management entity, contracts with individual physicians and assumes the responsibility of distributing PMPM payments.

PPO's are preferred provider organizations. A PPO is a line of business, like the HMO, that contracts at discounted rates with physicians, facility providers, and ancillary personnel. Unlike HMO's, PPO's retain financial risks. Some PPO's will perform their own precertification functions and pay claims as well as do their own utilization review. PPO's do not utilize PCP's as gatekeepers.

Under the PPO model, members can opt to see an in-network provider and receive a higher benefit level or may opt to see any out-of-network provider at a lower benefit level. Members can also self-refer to any specialist within the network.

PPO's generally have larger provider networks than HMO's and are less restrictive. Because they offer more flexibility than HMO's, the premiums paid for PPO's are typically higher than for HMO's.

Wait, we aren't finished with the alphabet soup. Other important initials await us, such as POS, or point of service; EPO's, or exclusive provider organizations; and PPA's, or preferred provider arrangements. To add to the confusion, we have had to learn to understand terms such as co-insurance and co-payments. Co-insurance is the percentage of the entire bill that the patient is responsible for paying after the deductible is met.

An example of co-insurance is when 90 percent of the payment will come from the managed-care company (in this case, generally a PPO), and the additional 10 percent will come from the member in the form of co-insurance.

Co-payments are flat amounts that are paid by the patient for a specific service provided. Co-payments are generally paid for physician office visits, ER visits, and various treatment services. The amount of the co-payment may be as little as five or ten dollars.

Doctors and hospitals have had to come to know a glossary of terms such as DRG's, discounted fee-for-service, case management, capitation, and risk contracting. The number of terms that now exist to manage the economics of medicine rivals the numbers of terms that define medical diseases themselves. It is virtually as important for a doctor to become as familiar with them as he is with the diseases he treats if he is to survive in today's new world.

Let's look at the basic definition of managed care: it is a mechanism by which a healthcare plan engages healthcare providers to provide quality medical care to a defined patient population in a cost-effective manner. By controlling costs and expenses, HMO's and PPO's are able to offer lower premiums to individuals and employer groups enrolled in their healthcare plans.

Part of controlling costs is by way of "negotiating" heavily discounted rates from both hospitals and physicians. Providers who don't adhere to cost containment or who don't agree to the reimbursement fees risk being locked out of the plan. In other words, the managed-care company will direct its patient base to the providers that offer the cheapest and most competitive rates while hopefully providing quality care.

Some of the positive aspects of the managed-care system are that hospitals and doctors are challenged with case managing each patient's hospital stay to lower the average length of hospitalization and to have patients go to a lower level of care as soon as medically feasible.

Doctors are expected to take care of their patients efficiently from both a medical and economic standpoint. Needless tests take up time, and time is money. Patients are discharged now sooner than they were ten years ago because doctors are held accountable for each day that a patient is hospitalized.

This is especially true with the system of DRG's that was invoked by HCFA for reimbursing hospitals for Medicare patients. Hospitals are paid the same for a given diagnosis no matter what the length of stay.

Case managers are trying to assist doctors in finding out-of-hospital solutions such as rehab centers, nursing homes, and skilled nursing units for their patients as soon as possible. The focus is on transferring patients from the acute hospital units to a lower level of care.

I have learned to start the preparations for my patients well in advance by conferring with social workers and case managers early in the hospital stay. They are extremely helpful and have bailed me out of trouble on many occasions when my options with patients seemed limited.

In some instances, costs are cut by shifting surgery from inpatient to outpatient facilities, called surgicenters, and in some instances cutting back on mental health care. In other instances, medical managers who review claims have flat out denied them, saying that they are unnecessary or too expensive.

Theoretically, managed care forces the issue of cost efficiency in the practice of medicine and is intended to maintain or improve quality. But does it really accomplish its intended purposes? And at what price and sacrifice? After all, the world is not perfect, and doctors are only human beings with human weaknesses.

In order to answer these questions, we must first examine the goals that we have for medical care in the new millennium. Depending on your perspective, the goals may vary, but I think there are certain basic goals that we as Americans, and as human beings, should share no matter what our background or profession.

Let me outline the goals that my years of medical practice have taught me are important and then let's examine whether managed care will help us attain them:

- The spiraling costs of health care need to be controlled, and healthcare costs should not bankrupt or destroy a person's life savings. The high, sometimes unreasonable, costs of health care are what caused managed care to be born in the first place. Affordable health care and prescription medication should be available to all Americans. Presently about forty million Americans are uninsured. Many more are partially insured because of the travesty of "preexisting illness" clauses that make a mockery of our current system of insurance coverage. These clauses pad the pockets of the insurers rather than protect the rights of millions of insured patients.
- We should strive to keep America on the cutting edge of medical education, research, and technological achievement and provide the best medical treatment possible. The quality of care should not be sacrificed to reduce costs.
- Providing better care for the aged and mentally ill is essential. We need to do better in both of these areas.
- We should strive for prevention of disease rather than concentrating on intervening once a disease has already occurred. Prevention is both cheaper in the long run and makes good common sense.
- Americans should have freedom of choice when it comes to choosing their physicians and other caregivers.
- We should not force people to wait unreasonable periods of time to obtain optimal medical care.
- Finally, there should be equality of care instead of the inequality that we have in our current system. Simply put, people who can afford insurance have access to

> better technology and testing than those who are poor. Some city health clinics cannot even budget for simple screening tests for many infectious diseases. There has to be some equality brought to a system that is based upon unequal access to essential healthcare needs.

Let's examine these goals in detail. I am sure that many of you are certain that there will be an automatic bias in my remarks because I am a physician. Please remember that I am also a patient as well as a baby boomer who would like to have a fair and efficient system in place when I get older.

Is medical care truly more affordable to Americans than it was in the pre-managed care era? The answer to this question on a superficial level is" yes," it is more affordable for some Americans—but not for all.

There is no question that decreased reimbursements to doctors and hospitals have led to the reduced cost of health care. There is also no question that some managed-care products offer cheaper and outwardly more attractive premiums than their older counterparts. But these premiums will probably rise if managed-care companies don't reap profits.

One has to wonder how much of the lower reimbursements to medical professionals are passed on to patients and how much to the managed-care bureaucracy itself. Don't forget that the managed-care companies have their own administrative costs as well, and they have to make a profit to stay in business.

Managed care has forced doctors to think about how best to treat a disease from a standpoint of economics. Hospitals work with doctors on a daily basis to find the ways to manage patients so as to improve their reimbursements.

This can include treating patients when feasible as outpatients rather than as inpatients, finding the diagnostic codes that can give the best payments, and transferring patients to skilled nursing units or to rehab as soon as possible.

In years past, doctors didn't have to give much thought about whether to admit or not to admit patients to the hospital.

It used to be routine to admit patients for comprehensive physicals or even minor medical ailments.

When I first started my practice, patients could expect to be admitted almost "on demand." To this day, patients still request to be admitted to the hospital for routine testing.

Forcing the doctor to think about cost-effective care is a good thing. Health care, no matter how good, should not be delivered haphazardly or in a fashion that would line the pockets of those who deliver it or who pay for it.

Medicare started the idea of reimbursing doctors and hospitals based upon diagnosis and treatment codes. Basically this meant that payment would be determined by what Medicare felt was reasonable for any given service provided. An operation would be paid a certain amount no matter how complicated it might become. Interestingly, however, doctors in certain areas might be paid at a higher rate than those in other geographic areas for providing the same service.

DRG's determine how much a hospital gets paid for a patient stay. This means that for a given diagnosis, the hospital would get paid a certain amount no matter how many procedures were done, what complications ensued, or how long a patient needs to stay in the hospital as a result of a complication.

Doctors have been pressured for years to get Medicare patients out of the hospital as quickly and efficiently as possible in order to help the hospital avoid financial loss. Managed care carried all this a few steps further. Now doctors have to justify to a third party everything that is done to their patients. This is called getting "preauthorization."

Preauthorization is time consuming and frustrating. After years of training, I have to rely on a person miles away to approve what I do, even if he or she can't spell the name of the illness that I am treating. My staff and I spend countless hours on the phone dialing 1-800 numbers in order to obtain permission to perform even the most basic of tests. A lot of doctors facetiously refer to these as "1-800 U R Out of Here" numbers. This takes valuable time away from patient care, but unless doctors cooperate and play the game by managed-care rules, our patients won't get the care that they need, and we won't get paid. I would rather spend more time with my patients and less time talking to an answering machine, since it is often hard to reach a "real" human being on the other end of the line. Obviously, if there is an emergency, I treat the patient first and worry about dialing phone numbers later.

After tests are approved, doctors are reimbursed what is felt to be "fair" by the insurance company. As a result of this process, some services are denied and not reimbursed at all. If a patient needs a mammogram and the insurance company doesn't agree, the patient has to pay for it out of pocket. This allows the insurance companies, rather than doctors who have trained for years, to establish the standards for medical care.

Patients and doctors are essentially at the mercy of the insurance industry. In the case of HMO's, specialists are often at the mercy of primary-care givers to get approval of procedures as minor as an electrocardiogram. Only recently have lawgivers made managed-care companies liable for their decisions and recommendations, and since then, at least one has decided to put these decisions in the hands of doctors instead of non-medical personnel.

The bottom line is that even though costs are superficially lower with managed care, other issues need to be examined closely, such as "quality of care." Certain tests and treatments may be denied without good reason.

A patients' rights bill was passed in Texas in 1997 that allows patients to appeal the decisions of their HMO's. Half of these appeals have been decided in favor of the patient. Physicians and medical associations are currently at the forefront of trying to pass a bill in Congress that should soon become national law. Not surprisingly, there has been active lobbying by the managed-care industry to prevent passage of a final bill that would protect patients' rights.

Since the passage of the patients' rights bill, there has been no increase in the number of uninsured patients, nor has there been an increased number of lawsuits against managed-care companies in Texas or in other states with similar legislation. The doom and gloom projections of the managed-care industry stating that the number of lawsuits, premiums, and uninsured patients would rise because of this legislation have not become reality. But, interestingly, it is not hard for doctors and their staffs to obtain approval for necessary tests since this legislation was passed.

We have to ask ourselves, "Are we getting less for less" in many situations, and is that what we really want? Some insurance plans have given doctors negative incentives for care, meaning that more money would be left for physicians in a pot at the end of the year if they spend less money on tests.

Is this the way we want to save money? Are we being "**pennywise and pound foolish**?"

Lawmakers who have supplied us with the answers about how to curb the spiraling costs of health care have thus far failed to do anything at all about some of the major reasons why costs have risen. There are huge hidden costs of health care that have so far been given only lip service by our lawmakers.

Doctors are the targets of exponentially increasing lawsuits, many of which are frivolous, and are given little or no protection from the harassment and fear of practicing medicine with a "legal" gun pointed at their heads. Malpractice insurance has risen tremendously, and for some high-risk specialties such as OB/GYN and Anesthesiology, these rates have become prohibitive and drastically increase overhead costs to a ridiculous level. Many people in rural and inner-city areas can't get necessary medical services, such as obstetrical care, because doctors can't afford the insurance premiums needed to provide these services!

Doctors are forced to practice in a defensive posture by a society that gives them no choice but to protect themselves from the constant threat of litigation. Doctors order more tests than are often necessary because of this ever-present fear. They literally can't afford to make mistakes or misdiagnose their patients.

Patients in today's society are educated and demand the latest technology, and they often voice dissatisfaction if it is not utilized in their care. Doctors are caught in the middle of a system that is trying to conserve money on the one hand and consumers who are demanding the latest technology on the other.

The costs of technology are staggering. The number of new tests is multiplying as I write this book. Doctors struggle to keep up with the latest and greatest and yet contain costs at the same time.

The costs of medicine suffer as more tests are ordered to make patients happy and prevent litigation. Society pressures doctors to be expert clinicians and cost conscious at the same time. This sounds rather wonderful and utopian but can be rather tricky because medicine is not an exact science, and sometimes multiple tests are necessary to make a diagnosis or prescribe treatment.

I try to practice medicine with both my head and my heart. Unfortunately, the reality of how our society operates often gets in the way of being able to do my best. Ultimately, fear will have to be removed from a doctor's mind; this requires a paradigm shift from free and open litigation to a more controlled malpractice environment. Society has to put an end to the open-hunting season against doctors for our entire system to work.

Managed care cannot address the entire problem of cost control, and until society changes its way of thinking, nothing will. Fortunately, the insurance industry can now be co-defenders in malpractice suits; formerly doctors were unfairly exposed to the entire risk. Talk about being hung out to dry!

The managed-care industry needs to be regulated, and a leash needs to be put on the legal profession to truly decrease the costs of health care to an acceptable level. Thus far, legislators have seen the need to regulate only the caregivers. Where is the logic in this, and who is becoming richer in this system? And who is becoming poorer?

"Quality of care" is a concern to everyone in our society. None of us wants to get the second-rate care that we fear from socialized medicine, and none of us wants America to lose its technological edge. But can we have our cake and eat it too?

There are no easy answers here. Managed care is definitely not the answer and doesn't assure us of being on the cutting edge of technology in the twenty-first century. If anything, it threatens to undermine our position of being world leaders in medical care.

America produces some of the best doctors in the world and is at the cutting edge of technology. The problem is that we do not know how to utilize our valuable resources, and we even put them at risk with our corporate-medicine environment.

Decreased reimbursements to teaching institutions have threatened the core of medical education in this country. Teaching hospitals, like all other hospitals in this country, are forced to look at the bottom line. Many programs are being slashed or cut, faculty positions are being decreased, and technology itself, which is not affordable, is threatened.

What long-term effects will this have on the training programs that produce some of the best doctors in the world? Medical-school applications have seen a drop as college students look at other options that give them more freedom with less frustration.

Technology is at risk as well. If a technological advancement is not reimbursed reasonably well, it will often be put on the back burner, even if it improves the quality of care that can be delivered. DRG rules for inpatient care mean that hospitals will be paid the same no matter what services are provided, so it is a harder fight for doctors to obtain some of the latest advances in technology.

When doctors go to hospital administrators with recommendations, they are asked if the equipment they are requesting will improve medical care, how much it will cost, and whether it is reimbursable and profitable for the hospital. It is important to look at equipment and services with a cost-benefit analysis.

Many doctors, again being human, try to allocate their time in a profitable manner. To maintain their income, some might increase the number of their procedures or spend less time with each patient in order to see a higher patient volume per day.

Higher patient and procedure volume are necessary to maintain a doctor's income in the managed-care era; it's simple arithmetic. Quality of care may suffer as a result, and patient satisfaction, in all likelihood, will drop. I have talked to many patients who feel "brushed off" by doctors who are trying to hurry and do as much as they can in the shortest period of time. Doctors are not paid by the minute.

The future of medicine likely will see the centralization of technology in a few institutions that are designated centers of excellence by insurance companies. That doesn't mean that everyone else outside is a mediocre provider, but that these centers would be able to provide the services at a lower cost and perhaps more efficiently.

I have major concerns with an insurance industry that looks for the cheapest but not necessarily the best contractor and that limits the number of doctors on a panel, often utilizing a first-come,-first-served basis so that patients often have to change doctors and lose continuity of care.

Continuity of care is extremely important both to quality and to patient satisfaction. A lot of patient dissatisfaction relates to the loss of choices in both the patient's care and his or her caregiver. In our current system, it is difficult for patients to have inexpensive care with low premiums and still have freedom of choice and the input into their care that they have had in the past.

Marcia Angell, M.D., eloquently expressed the current situation in a recently published editorial in *The New England Journal of Medicine:*

"What we should instead conclude is that the private managed care market has been a miserable failure at delivering health care. It has creamed off ever larger percentages of health care premiums in bloated administrative and marketing costs and profits, it has rewarded health plans that cherry-pick the healthy and avoid the sick, and it has resisted at every turn providing adequate services to those unfortunate enough to need them."[10]

One of the major inequalities in our system is its inability to provide adequate economic support for the aged and mentally ill. An all too frequent dilemma is exemplified by the plight of a senior citizen who lives on social security and cannot afford to pay for his or her medication. My office is constantly providing samples (that we obtain from the drug industry) for patients and trying to find cheaper medications as substitutes for high-priced brand-name medicines that people simply can't afford.

There are countless patients that I have been forced to hospitalize with acute illnesses that were exacerbated by their inability to afford their medications. One of the best preventive measures our society can take to avoid illness and decrease the costs of health care is to ensure that the average person can get his or her medications at reasonable cost and still be able to afford to eat. A choice between paying for groceries and paying for medications should never have to be made.

"Chronically ill, older Americans may thus be hit with annual drug costs of many thousands of dollars—sums they simply cannot pay. There are frequent stories of older Americans who play out

their prescriptions for as long as possible by taking reduced doses, share drugs with their spouses, or simply do without, choosing food and heat over drugs.

Medicare recipients with no supplementary insurance pay on average twice as much for the 10 most commonly prescribed drugs as do favored customers, such as large HMO's and the Veterans Affairs system."[11]

The chief culprits in this horror story are the government and the drug industry itself. Our government needs to provide prescription relief as soon as possible for its Medicare beneficiaries, most who are on fixed incomes. There is no excuse for Americans to have to pay a higher price for drugs than their counterparts throughout the world—often twice as much as Europeans and Canadians for the same drug.[12]

Drugs are priced higher here in America to ostensibly offset research and development costs and to adjust for our higher standard of living. We need to find ways to decrease the costs of medications here in America, even if it means less profit for the drug industry. Surprisingly, there has been little regulation of this important player in the costs and delivery of health care. It is hard to justify the costs of drugs to Americans when we stop and realize that the pharmaceutical industry has been the most profitable industry in the United States.

"According to a recent issue of *Fortune*, in 1999 the pharmaceutical industry realized on average an 18.6% return on revenues. Commercial banking was second, at 15.8%, and other industries ranged from 0.5 to 12.1%."[13]

This appears superficially to be a case of "the rich getting richer and the poor getting poorer," but it's far more than that. This situation is a threat to human life and needs to change.

As a physician, I love the fact that new drugs are available that help me wage war against disease, but I also see tremendous inequality in the availability of these wonderful drugs to the rich and to the poor. I also see a tremendous amount of redundancy in the drugs that are made available to physicians, and not all of them are necessary. The majority of them certainly aren't cheap.

How do we decide how much a pill should cost or how much money should be allocated for research and development of new drugs? I feel guilty asking my patients to take pills that cost more than an entire day's worth of food.

The pharmaceutical industry is a runaway train with a conductor on Wall Street and quite a few lobbyists in Washington:

> **"The pharmaceutical industry is under mounting scrutiny because of rapidly increasing expenditures for drugs in the United States. Drug expenditures are now the fastest growing component of health care costs, increasing at the rate of 15% per year. They account for eight percent of health care spending, and at their current rate of increase, they will soon surpass spending for physicians' services and, for many health maintenance organizations (HMO's), the costs of hospitalization."**[14]

Medicare is full of inconsistencies and inefficiency. In a weird twist of logic, Medicare pays doctors less if they do several procedures on one day than if they do them over several days; for example, if I do a heart catheterization and an angioplasty on the same day, Medicare reimburses me less than if I do them on consecutive or different days!

Obviously, this policy indirectly encourages doctors to perform their procedures over longer periods of time and even to prolong hospital stays (which ultimately increases costs). Hopefully, doctors will do what's necessary and practical for their patients, but where is the logic in a system that rewards doctors for taking care of their patients over longer periods of time and pays them less for multiple procedures done in emergency situations?

A lot of patients who are employed have no health insurance. I hope that employers will receive more incentive to insure their workers in the form of tax credits and other subsidies from the government. Employees should receive tax credits that are inversely related to their income so that low-income workers can afford health insurance. Many of our uninsured are poor and cannot afford even basic coverage provided by their employers.

Both employers and employees should be given economic incentive to obtain something so vitally important as health insurance. It is well known that people without insurance tend to delay seeking medical attention until they are so sick that they must be hospitalized. At this stage, their healthcare expenses drain our system even further, validating the argument that it would be cost effective to help people to obtain both insurance and prescription drugs to prevent illness from occurring in the first place. Let's face the facts: Intervention is more expensive than prevention, and it is more painful to our economy and to our patients!

It is possible that employers may drop healthcare coverage if premiums get any higher, as is predicted by some. As managed-care expenses go up, they are passed on to the employers who pass them on in turn to the employees. Something has "to give."

Hopefully, health insurance companies will drop "preauthorization" completely. It is expensive, a nuisance to doctors, and very inefficient for patient care. The decision-making needs to be placed in the hands of doctors, where it belongs; it doesn't belong in the hands of insurance companies with a conflict of interest because of a desire to both save and make money.

There are no easy answers. Holding the insurance industry accountable for its actions is a first step. Streamlining of the system is essential to make it more friendly and efficient for everyone to use. Regulation of the legal profession and drug industries is necessary to further lower the costs of health care and to fulfill the goals that I have previously outlined. So far, lawmakers have only concentrated on regulating doctors, which is the simplest thing to do.

By and large, doctors have little or no recourse when faced with these rules and regulations. They are often too busy to organize within their own ranks, and they tend to be independent creatures. One doctor described organizing doctors as being a lot like "herding a bunch of cats." They tend to do their own thing and look out for themselves instead of each other.

As a society, we need to ask ourselves if we can truly buy a Cadillac for the price of a motor scooter without losing quality.

Our system is broken, and until we figure out the right answers, we had better learn the dance called:

The HMO Shuffle

Have you heard about that new HMO?

The doctors are good, but the referrals

Are slow.

By the way, that great doctor of yours for

Fifteen years,

Isn't on our list—better switch gears!
Instead, better call your PCP.
He hasn't been around too long,
But he's agreed to a minimal fee.

If you have problems, you could always switch
To a PPO.
You won't need a PCP, but the answer's still
"no!"

Your doctor will work harder for a lot
Less money.
To him, the steps of the shuffle are not
Very funny.

Best learn to sidestep quickly, and don't be
A quitter.
Your body was just sold to the
Lowest bidder.

"Truth Bypasses"—A Doctor's Dilemma

Doctors are caught between doing what is best for their patients and dealing with managed care and governmental regulations.

I have often thought that my patient would benefit from an extra day in the hospital only to find that someone sitting at a desk light years away had not only decided that the extra day was unnecessary and unimportant but decided to tell my patient that what I was doing was both improper and too expensive.

That point is the moment of decision, the moment of truth. Do I go against the grain of years of experience and discharge the patient, or do I "fudge the truth" on the chart and do what I feel is the right thing for my patient? This has become known as "gaming the system."

This is a dilemma that poses many questions about the ethics of being a doctor who is morally bound as his patient's caregiver and yet at the same time is obligated to a system that goes against everything that he has learned as a doctor and threatens the welfare of his patients.

According to an article published in the *Journal of the American Medical Association*,[15] a random survey of 720 doctors nationwide in 1998 showed that 39 percent used one of several tactics:

- Exaggerating the severity of an illness to help patients avoid being discharged early from the hospital.
- Reporting inaccurate diagnoses on bills.
- Reporting non-existent symptoms to secure insurance coverage for testing.

A big part of the problem is that doctors are caught in the middle of the demands of the patient on the one hand and the restrictions of the insurance industry on the other. Deception is a quiet way that some doctors may be voicing their protest against a system that they feel has gone haywire and is unfair to them and to their patients:

> **"Physicians are thus caught in 2 sets of conflicting demands. Legally, physicians are contractually bound to adhere to reimbursement policies yet are also liable for failure to deliver an equally high standard of care to all patients, regardless of ability to pay. Ethically, physicians are caught between the compelling principles of social justice on the one hand and beneficence, or mercy, on the other."[16]**

There is no excuse for lying about what we do as doctors. But the system sometimes leaves us no choice if we are to truly be our patients' advocates. **A gentle stretching of the truth** is sometimes just what the doctor ordered. At crucial moments, it is necessary to fight fire with fire.

"Big Brother" Is Watching

You are probably beginning to understand why most doctors don't particularly enjoy practicing medicine in the world of managed care. The deluge of paperwork is nearly insurmountable. The costs of running an office and being compliant with the current system make it very difficult to practice independently outside of a clinic setting where that responsibility is assumed by corporate professionals who are paid to do the paperwork and to negotiate the contracts. Big corporations are a lot more powerful negotiating contracts at the bargaining table than I can be by myself as a solo practitioner.

It's amazing how much time my office staff spends on the phone and filling out the paperwork that is required to keep up with the demands of managed care. I have had to drastically increase my office staff to deal with these mind-boggling problems and the confusion it has produced. Often I have had to get on the phone myself to try to sort out the mess; most of the time, I am on hold while I am trying to find the right person to talk to. Managed care has given birth to unmanageable chaos.

I have been an independent practitioner for seventeen years, and it is becoming harder and harder to deal with the business and medical ends of my practice at the same time. I can understand why more and more doctors are deciding that they need to make a change into a different environment or even into another profession. Job dissatisfaction is rampant, and I have heard many doctors talk a lot about "life after medicine."

A lot of doctors are afraid for their survival and are essentially running scared. Patients can be lost overnight with the signing of a contract. I have personally lost hundreds of patients because managed-care contracts were signed with another group of doctors in town. The result can decimate a practice, even an established one like mine. There are times when I am not sure whether my practice can survive until I am old enough to retire. I feel powerless when I see patients whom I have known for years, and to whom I have become attached, having no choice but to see other doctors.

Recently a long-term patient of mine was forced to switch from one insurer to another because of financial reasons. He sadly informed me that he could not come back to see me again. It was hard to say goodbye, and it left me depressed. He also regretted leaving, but he felt he had no choice. This is a scene that is played out all too regularly in my office and, I am sure, in the offices of almost every doctor in this country.

I am also afraid that if I don't practice medicine in a way that is deemed cost efficient, then I may be in jeopardy of being dropped by insurance companies in the future. I know that my outcomes are constantly being monitored by both hospitals and regulatory agencies. I am being judged not only on my clinical abilities but also on whether I spend more money than Doctor "X" down the road.

It's not enough that hospitals now tell us how much money we are making or losing for them; we also have to worry about whether or not we are doing enough procedures to maintain our licenses.

In the future, regulatory agencies more than likely will require doctors to do specific numbers of cases to maintain their credentials. You know where that leads? Of course, it leads to doctors doing unnecessary procedures to get the numbers necessary to be deemed "proficient."

Have no doubt: "Big Brother" is watching. Medicine has become "big business." No physician that I know feels secure in today's managed-care environment. From my own personal standpoint, I know that I went into medicine to help people, not to have someone constantly tell me how and when to do it.

I had no idea that insurance companies and lawyers would dictate so much of how I went about my job. I came to the realization that I went into the most regulated field in America today outside of the military. From my own personal standpoint, I went into medicine to help people, not to have someone tell me how, when, and where to do it and then pay me what he or she thinks I'm worth—or not pay me at all..

Big Brother has taken some of the fun and satisfaction out of practicing medicine, and it is downright frustrating at times because I like what I do, and I want to do it right.

Be on the Lookout for Space Invaders

I have learned to know the fourth alligator well. He is a space invader and represents demands on my time that exceed even my wildest dreams. I have a beeper that follows me into the most private moments of my life; I can't even go to the bathroom in peace! I take calls during the wee hours of the morning and late at night. I have to admit that there are times when I have problems falling back to sleep, even after all these years. I feel too stimulated from the adrenaline surge to be able to "turn it on" and then suddenly "shut it off."

I now have at least three ways that people can awaken me at night. There is the beeper, the phone by my bed, and the old-fashioned knock on the door. The phone line went out one night, and my answering service went crazy trying to find me. They even sent the police to my house! People panic when they can't reach me. It feels good to be needed, but enough is enough!

People can also find me by fax and by e-mail. The only way to truly "get away from it all" is to get out of town, and then the demands still follow me if there are problems in the office or with my practice. I always arrange for another doctor to "cover for me," but I still have the ultimate responsibility of taking care of my patients twenty-four hours a day, seven days a week.

When I first went into medicine, I was compulsive and was actually enamored by this lifestyle. The phone calls made me tired but were part of the job. I didn't really mind having little privacy, and it felt great to be needed. I essentially became numb to the demands of the profession that I had chosen, and having "**no life**" just became my normal life.

I have learned to cherish my privacy because there is so little of it, and after almost eighteen years of doctoring, my priorities have changed. I now need peace and solitude for my own well-being. Status symbols don't matter quite as much as they used to. I have learned to protect my quiet time and my space.

Time off is not taken for granted after years of working long hours, holidays, and weekends. My mind and my body have paid a toll for this hard work. Hard work doesn't come free of charge, like I used to think when I was younger.

Over the years, I have learned the importance of that simple word that I have repeated so often in this book, the word "**no.**"

It has been a hard word to say because, as a doctor, I have wanted to "be there" for everyone at anytime.

Now I look out for my own happiness, not just as a physician but also as a human being. I can sense when I am being used and abused, and I have learned to somewhat selfishly protect myself from space invaders. The result of not protecting myself has been "burnout," which will be discussed in other sections of this book.

Sometimes strangers or people off the street come to my office or home wanting to talk to me during my office hours or during time with my family. It became important to set limits for myself and for others. I truly want to help people, but sometimes there isn't enough of me to go around. I can't be a doctor 24/7/365.

There are times when I feel like everyone wants a "piece of the rock." Cloning myself is not an option. Helping others can be not only exhilarating and rewarding but also a draining experience—that is, if I allow it to be.

The worst space invader is definitely not human. It is a little box that chirps and vibrates when it wants to get your attention. It follows me into the bathroom, restaurants, and movie theatres. It pulls me away from showers, eating, and intimate moments. It is technically called a beeper, but I have thought of many other names for it, most of which are unprintable here.

I have wanted to throw it away, stomp on it, scream at it, and even flush it down the commode, but it has survived until this day. It is an albatross around my waist and makes me feel like a modern-day version of the ancient mariner.

Sometimes I just want to retreat into the solitude of my own world. It's easy to lose track of who and what you are in all this chaos. My son just asked me for a beeper for his birthday. My initial response was, "Are you really sure you want this?" I wish I could teach him to be wary of space invaders, but he will just have to learn on his own, just as I did:

Overstimulation

Beeper at my left, cell phone to my right,
E-mail in front of me,
Relentlessly stalking me, day and night
Where is peace and tranquility?
Beeping…chirping…ringing….
Futilely,
I seek serenity with all my might!

It took me years to overcome my compulsive nature and realize that there really is such a thing as an “on-off” button. This switch is a key to my door of sanity.

False Expectations

The last alligator is not in the picture at all but is perhaps the most dangerous and most insidious troublemaker of the whole lot. He is sly and instigates the other alligators into doing his dirty work.

Behind many of a doctor’s problems are false expectations, not just from patients but also from society in general, even from myself! I am expected to be constantly available, to do perfect or near perfect work, and save money for managed-care companies and hospitals at the same time. Sometimes, I am expected to be the hero or the knight on the white horse coming to the rescue.

I am expected to know all the answers and to work tirelessly for the benefit of humanity. I am expected to sacrifice a lot of my life for the sake of others and still be in a good mood, even when I am exhausted or sick.

Doctors are public figures; especially in small towns. I frequently run into my patients when I go out shopping or to a restaurant. Sometimes I get a courteous, "Hello, you remember me, don't you?"

Often I hear, "Dr. Farber, I know you haven't seen me in a few years, but do you remember that medication that you put me on? You know, it's giving me all kinds of problems. What do you think I should do about it? And by the way, tell me about those test results, won't you? What do you think is really wrong with me?"

Sometimes I also hear, "Doctor, I can't believe you're eating that juicy steak!" I have often thought about wearing sunglasses, especially in restaurants, so that people can't see if I "practice what I preach."

People often surprise me by what they expect me to remember about their own particular medical problems when I see so many patients every day. But then again, most people are the center of their own universe.

Surprisingly, a lot of people think that I want to talk medicine twenty-four hours a day! They really must think that a doctor has no life outside of medicine. I learned to politely tell people that it is great seeing them but that I can't really discuss their test results or their case very well without their charts. "Please call me at the office" is my firm but friendly response.

I also feel an overwhelming sense of responsibility for my patients because I am supposed to be there for them. Deep down, I feel that I am the best doctor for many of them because I know them so well. But in reality, it is just hard to "let go" because this requires knowing that I am not indispensable. My expectations from myself are sometimes the biggest thorn in my side.

And then there are attorneys who expect doctors to make mistakes because they know that no one is perfect. At least they are realistic and know we are human.

Some people probably can't understand how a doctor could become so cynical.

Postscript: Did the Duck "Get Away from It All?"

Well, our friendly protagonist has survived so far. There is still a smile on his face. He still enjoys life and has learned to keep the alligators at a safe distance.

The good news is that the alligators are just nuisances along the way that can be either tamed or ignored. It's just a matter of learning how to outsmart them in order to "*Get Away from It All.*"

For all of the negatives that I have talked about, medicine is still the most rewarding profession in the world. I realize that God has led me through trials and tribulations to become a better person and a better doctor and to realize a more fully enjoyable life.

Above all else, my life has been a learning process that has taught me to have both patience and a sense of humor. Now it is time to talk about the people who have taught me the most: my patients.

Endnotes

1. Rice, "How Plaintiff's Lawyers Pick Their Targets," *Medical Economics*, April 2000, p. 96.

2. Ibid., p. 104.

3. Ibid., p. 106.

4. *Webster's New World College Dictionary, Third Edition* (Simon and Schuster, Inc.), 1996.

5. Kohn, et al., *To Err Is Human: Building a Safer Health System* (Washington, D.C.: National Academy Press), 2000.

6. Brennan, "The Institute of Medicine Report on Medical Errors—Could It Do Harm?" *New England Journal of Medicine*, Vol. 342, No. 15, April 13, 2000, p. 1123.

7. Angres and Talbott, *Healing the Healer, The Addicted Physician* (Madison, Connecticut, Psychosocial Press, 1998) p. 109.

8. Ibid., p. 119.

9. Covey, *The 7 Habits of Highly Effective Families* (Golden Books, Franklin Covey Company), 1997.

10. Angell, "Patients' Rights Bills and other Futile Gestures," *New England Journal of Medicine*, Vol. 342, No. 22, June 1, 2000.

11. Angell, "The Pharmaceutical Industry—To Whom Is It Accountable?" *New England Journal of Medicine*, Vol. 342, No. 25, June 22, 2000.

12. Ibid.

13. Ibid.

14. Ibid., p. 1903.

15. Wynia, et al., "Physician Reimbursement Rules for Patients—Between a Rock and a Hard Place, *Journal of the American Medical Association*, Vol., 283, No. 14, April 12, 2000.

16. Ibid.

CHAPTER 5

The Doctor's "Eleventh Commandment"

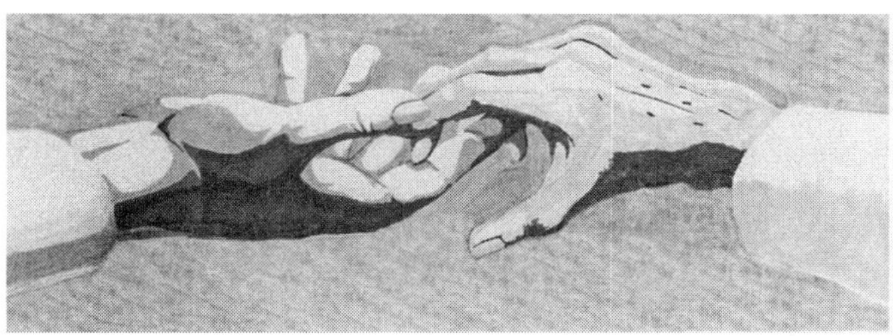

"Like a bridge over troubled water, I will lay me down."

"Bridge Over Troubled Water," Simon and Garfunkel

There is nothing as sacred to the medical profession as the relationship between a doctor and his patient. It is the sun around which everything else revolves, and it gives light to a doctor's universe. It is the very essence, heart, and soul of a doctor's reason for being. Forget the bullshit of dealing with malpractice suits, managed care, and the Internal Revenue Service. This is what being a doctor is all about! My patients are the reasons why I am still doing what I am doing.

A robot could probably be taught to diagnose and treat a patient, but it could never be taught to be a doctor who feels empathy for others. I know some doctors have been accused of being robot-like because they treat the disease and forget about the person who has the disease. The doctor-patient relationship, like most other relationships, is not always easy.

As technology evolves, we risk losing sight of some very basic fundamental values that are timeless. In spite of the passing of millenniums, some important ideas and beliefs have never changed, and heaven help us if they do.

The Ten Commandments are still as fundamentally important today as they were when Moses delivered them from Mount Sinai. Certain values should and will remain essential to our survival. Although I will not be presumptuous enough to compare anything to the values that God handed down to the children of Israel, I feel so strongly about the covenant between doctor and patient that I have termed this covenant, **The Doctor's "Eleventh Commandment."**

A covenant is a sacred promise. A doctor's relationship with his patients brings with it certain specific promises, expectations, and burdens, just like a marriage. The purpose of this chapter is to discuss the issues that define this relationship and what makes this relationship, in a real sense, "sacred."

Doctors have been looked upon by patients as advocates for their physical needs for thousands of years. They are the "safe harbors" that patients are looking for in times of distress and pain. The trust that patients place in their doctors is not unlike the trust that is placed in a rabbi or minister, and the prayers that are said in hospital beds are just as powerful as if they were said in churches or synagogues.

Like Simon and Garfunkel say in their famous song, some people are a "bridge over troubled water" to ease the minds and physical suffering of others. Doctors are such people. And they are there even when no one else is to be found, when people are all alone in the world.

This chapter is dedicated to my patients.

A Doctor's Covenants with His Patients

When a doctor agrees to take care of a patient, he morally agrees to certain "marriage vows" or promises. Why are these so important? In my experience, a doctor can maintain a better relationship with his patients if he follows certain rules or "codes of conduct." I am not trying to preach and tell doctors how to practice medicine or conduct their lives, but I think they will serve themselves and their patients better if they take these promises seriously.

The first vow is one of confidentiality. Nothing about the patient's condition should be discussed with anyone else, even the patient's immediate family, without proper consent. The exception, of course, is if the patient is incapacitated mentally, is comatose, or is a minor. Family and friends will try to test this basic doctrine and ask you probing questions to get information. It is important to remember that the patient may not want other people to know even simple things about his or her condition.

Doctors ask many personal questions in order to obtain a diagnosis, and the answers should stay confidential. It is not unlike attorney-client privilege or the privacy of a confessional. The questions and answers should both be made in good faith and without fear of retribution or punishment. Patients may confess things to doctors out of fear, things that other people should not know, sometimes things that could get them into trouble with their spouse or even with the law.

The second vow is to do everything possible to ease pain and suffering without prejudice. A patient's financial status, race, color, or creed should not interfere with that obligation. Nor should the nature of the disease affect the care.

Healthcare workers shouldn't avoid AIDS patients, but that is not always the reality. Doctors and nurses are afraid of exposure to this deadly virus, and they sometimes refuse to take care of patients with AIDS, which some consider the modern-day plague. Like the rest of society, they sometimes show prejudice towards those who are afflicted with diseases such as AIDS.

Patients should not be treated differently if they are uninsured or poor. That is not the way the system is currently set up. Doctors do a lot for poor people, but they can only touch the surface. Government policies need to assure everyone of equal care. This is the "for richer, for poorer" part of the vow.

A third vow for the doctor is to help the patient to live with dignity and to allow him to die with dignity. The goal is not necessarily to prolong life. "Death with dignity" is such an intense and hotly debated topic that it will be discussed further in a different section.

We need to allow the patient dignity both in life and in death. We do that by both knowing what his wishes are and by honoring them to the best of our abilities. It cannot be done without personal and deliberate communication. A part of this vow is to help the patient to not be a burden to those around him, but that does not mean that a doctor should be allowed to assist a patient in committing suicide. Allowing a patient who is terminal to die the way he wishes is very different from helping him to die.

The vow of "abstinence" is one that you shouldn't have to be a priest or monk to understand. It is incredibly important because we are all "human" and can be attracted to each other on many levels. Doctors and their patients are no exception. However, doctors need to be very careful about showing their "human side" at inappropriate times.

Patients come to the doctor looking for the relief of pain and suffering. They are extremely vulnerable at these times. The doctor-patient relationship is a lot like that of a parent to his child or a shepherd to his flock. It is important to remember how dependent children are for answers and protection. By allowing themselves to have anything more than platonic relationships with patients, doctors run the risk of abusing the trust placed in them and of taking advantage of patients who are vulnerable to emotional attachment when they are in pain and need objective guidance.

Physicians are objects of emotional and even physical attachment because of their position of power. Power is a tantalizing seductress to many people, especially when they are vulnerable. It can be an aphrodisiac to the strongest among us, but its effects can lead to disaster. Why? There are several reasons.

It is almost impossible for doctors to maintain clear medical judgment that is critical for decision-making when they have strong emotional bonds or physical intimacy with those under their care. Whenever I have tried to treat my loved ones, it has usually led to a biased opinion or one based on emotion rather than objectivity. This is certainly not in their best interests.

Doctors need to be very careful about casual flirtation because seemingly innocent actions can be misinterpreted. I love to hug my patients, and I am a very "touchy, feely" person. That is my nature. Usually my older patients are disappointed if they don't get their hugs and proper amount of TLC.

There is a problem, however. In today's climate of litigation, it is in vogue to sue people for sexual harassment. Doctors who act inappropriately with their patients or fellow professionals leave themselves exposed to this allegation. Unless a nurse or aide is in the room, it is "your word against theirs." It's a "no-win" situation that no doctor wants.

I have a word of caution and advice for a doctor who decides to pursue intimacy with a patient. It is certainly your right but get another doctor for your patient! Even that may not prevent you from being sued in the future if you maintain the relationship. Ask yourself if this is real emotion and affection or just living a fantasy and an attraction.

A very important promise that a doctor makes to his patients is to treat them with honesty and sincerity whether it is about test results, the illness or its prognosis, or even the bill. If a mistake is made, then it is best to confess to it rather than hiding it or sweeping it under the rug. I have found that patients are generally intelligent and appreciate honesty. Usually they understand "honest mistakes."

People are generally forgiving by nature. However, if a patient discovers that he or she was lied to or deceived in any aspect of care, watch out! The road to litigation is paved with people's perceptions of arrogance and dishonesty. When doctors are afraid to admit the truth, they invite malpractice suits. Sometimes doctors are afraid to admit that they don't know everything. Society wants them to be experts.

Just a note on "perception" to reiterate what I have said in the previous chapter: It is the patient's perception of his or her care that is important, not necessarily the actual care received. If a doctor is not straightforward with his patients, then he may be perceived as trying to hide something. Most doctors want to be honest with their patients, but they don't know how to communicate very well and therefore make themselves look like they are hiding something and not being forthright.

The last vow that I would like to discuss is the vow of "fidelity." Fidelity here means loyalty to your patients. Doctors should never put themselves in a situation that creates a conflict of interest with their patients' welfare.

Insurance companies test this loyalty when they give doctors incentives for doing less work on their patients. "More is less" here, and this system leads to poor medical care. I cringe when I hear that doctors are being given financial rewards for ordering fewer tests on their patients. A system with "kickbacks" has no place in medicine and should be outlawed. It pits doctors against their patients' interests!

Trust—The Basic Building Block

"Real Communication Happens When People Feel Safe"[1]

Trust is the basic building block of the doctor-patient relationship, just as it is in any interpersonal relationship. It is a by-product of feeling safe with the person who you are with or talking to. It isn't acquired overnight. Trust sometimes takes months or years to acquire. That is why the effects of managed care are so sad. It helps to destroy what took hard work and time to build. You strive to prove that you are not only good at what you do but that you are truthful and compassionate as well. Then managed care sweeps that rug out from under you.

Trust needs to go in both directions, and it is important for a doctor to be able to trust that his patients will be loyal and believe in him, unless, of course, he does something to violate the contract between them. Patients need to have faith that everything that a doctor does is for their benefit and that there is absolute confidentiality.

Without this trust, you might as well throw away everything that a doctor learns in medical school because it doesn't matter.

Allowing People to "Ventilate"

People often hear what they want to hear and don't really listen to what I tell them. One of the earliest phases of dealing with grief is denial. Another is anger. Both denial and anger can make a doctor's job of communicating very challenging. Having family members present with the patient during important conversations sometimes eliminates miscommunication and gives support to the patient at an important time.

Allowing the patient to ventilate frustrations and speak openly doesn't always guarantee that they are listening with an open mind or comprehending what is being said. Denial is a powerful barrier to communication. Frustration and anger lead to misunderstandings, which then lead to hard feelings.

It is important to allow patients to talk uninterrupted, if at all possible, about their feelings. Unfortunately, a doctor's day is seldom without multiple interruptions. Sometimes I may receive five or six phone calls while I am trying to talk with one patient. It is difficult for me to listen attentively if I am preoccupied or fatigued. I try my best to set aside interruptions when I am facing an important conversation. This saves me time in the long run, and the patient appreciates it.

There have been numerous times in my years of practice when I thought that I communicated my ideas or intentions to a patient only to have discovered later that I was totally misunderstood. At times, this has been my fault and at times the result of medications that cause temporary amnesia. Sometimes people just don't listen because they are preoccupied. Enlisting the family's support can prevent this problem. This is crucial at difficult emotional times, and it supports the doctor as much as the patient.

Basically, doctors have an obligation to their patients to give them all of the facts that are necessary in order to make informed decisions, even if these facts make them uncomfortable. No doctor likes to give a patient or family bad news, but sugarcoating the truth doesn't do patients any favors and can lead to later resentment. They need to know the truth so that they can plan for the future, whether it is good or bad.

Empathy and the Art of Medicine

The doctor-patient relationship is what the art of medicine is all about. Relating to people is not something easily teachable, and some doctors are naturally better at it than others. And unfortunately, medical school offers precious little training in this important area.

We need to talk on a patient's level, and preferably eye-to-eye, so that he or she can have a better chance of understanding what we are saying. Being a patient myself has aided tremendously my ability to communicate and empathize with patients. I am convinced that we would have better and more understanding doctors if we occasionally had to walk in our patients' footsteps and swallow our own medicine. Doctors need to "walk the walk," not just "talk the talk!"

Perhaps the password in the doctor-patient relationship is empathy. Understanding not only the meaning of this word but also how to apply it will prevent physicians from acting in ways that allow other people to perceive them as being cruel and unfeeling. It is not only "what we say but also how we say it" that is important. Crucial conversations cannot be rushed, and we need to make our patients understand that we feel for what they are going through and will help them through it anyway possible.

Sometimes the wrong person may break bad news at the wrong moment. I had a very ill cardiac patient who was told that he needed a transplant by a cardiologist who was "covering" for me over the weekend. The patient resented hearing the news from him instead of me, and hearing it in that manner made the patient dislike him and wonder why I had not been honest before.

My sin of omission had been equated with dishonesty. It is hard to predict what other people will say and do that might unintentionally interfere with my relationship with my patients. Sometimes a well-meaning, seemingly innocuous comment will trigger a reaction of anger. The take-home message for me is that I needed to not only communicate better with my patients but also with my colleagues and staff because they represent me.

Empathy is critical in allowing a doctor to think about how to word things appropriately in sensitive situations. I can usually tell when my patients are becoming frightened and when they have lost hope. I cannot prevent fear or any human emotion, but I can certainly try to keep my patients from losing something as precious as their hope for recovery or survival.

There are few situations where I feel that there is nothing at all that I can do to help patients who come to me with their problems, even if it is just giving them a better quality of life for as long as possible. It is usually possible to instill some hope without losing sight of reality.

Patients tend to do better if they are not deprived of the feeling that they have a potential to enjoy other people and the world around them. It is an essential part of their treatment and an essential need of the human spirit. Pessimism and depression are natural during illness but can be negatives when it comes to getting well. It's only logical.

Attitude and perseverance have a lot to do with a patient's recovery and prognosis. I have found that the people who are able to fight their diseases effectively are those who think positively and are willing to work hard in their own behalf. They know that I can't do it all for them.

They are the ones who work hard in their smoking cessation and rehabilitation programs and who exercise and follow their diets. They see themselves and their problems in a positive light and generally work hard to be well.

I once entered a hospital room and asked one of my patients how he felt that day. He responded that he felt rather "low" and seemed discouraged. I talked with him for several minutes and told him that I felt encouraged and that he had made progress. I made it clear that I had a goal to send him home as soon as possible, but I didn't know when that would be.

Just hearing that I had a goal for him perked him up. When I finished talking, it was obvious that he was not about to give up. He felt motivated by a few simple words. These words were not meant to give him unrealistic hope but to give him encouragement and incentive to wake up the next morning and try as hard as he could. His fear had been that he would never make it home.

It is not hard to detect fear and anger in patients if one has sensitivity to their needs. Sometimes fear and anger wind up getting directed towards me because I am the doctor. I become an easy and accessible target, "the fall guy," especially if I am the bearer of bad news. Some of it is misdirected at my office personnel or other healthcare workers.

These are natural emotions of the ill and are best responded to with compassion and understanding. That is not always easy, and sometimes I have to make a concerted effort to restrain my own anger at times. I am human, and sometimes I also need to ventilate out of frustration or fatigue. I try to remember what it is like to be a patient in order to avoid confrontations.

If—as Stephen Covey puts it so well—I first "**seek to understand before being understood**,"[2] I can usually calm an angry patient. If I sense that she is angry with me, I have sometimes even asked her directly if this is the case and, if so, why. If a patient knows that you will listen when she talks to you, she will form a bond with you that will survive most any ordeal and make the relationship a satisfying one for both of you.

Despite its inherent difficulties, the doctor-patient relationship is not only the most important but also the most rewarding aspect of being a doctor. As you will see later, my relationships with my patients have provided me with insight and fulfillment that have made me both a better person and a better doctor.

What Are the Patient's Responsibilities in the Doctor-Patient Relationship?

Most avenues are two-way streets, and the doctor-patient relationship is no exception.

There has to be some common meeting ground and some mutual give and take to achieve the goals that both desire. These goals may be different for different situations; for some it might be achieving a cure, for others, improving the quality of life, and for even others, living out their last days as free of pain as possible at home with their family.

These goals should be defined as early as possible and strategies or plans of action, devised and implemented to achieve the desired results. There are highly effective strategies that doctors can utilize, and they will be discussed in a later chapter.

What are a patient's responsibilities in this relationship? The answer quite simply is that no strategy will work unless the patient adopts the attitude that he or she is a major instrument of his or her own success or failure. Doctors can't shoulder that responsibility by themselves.

Let's talk about the responsibilities that a patient has to both himself and to his or her physician.

First, it is important to keep scheduled appointments. I know this sounds pretty ridiculous, but it is amazing how many people will postpone their doctors' appointments because they need to get their hair done or, even better, because they feel "too sick to go the doctor!" I have heard all sorts of excuses over the years. Some people have even cancelled their appointments with me because they want to get their nails done! Many people put their own care on the back burner and just find more important things to do.

A patient needs to tell her physician how she feels, including how medications are affecting her. She needs to be honest and upfront about personal situations in her life that are causing stress. Withholding information is dangerous and makes the doctor's job very difficult. Misinformation is worse than no information at all!

An "honest effort" on their own behalf is all that I ask from my patients. And I ask them to try not to undermine what we are trying to accomplish by being noncompliant with their regimen. But then again, I can't force a patient to swallow their pills or to take my advice. I talk, explain, and try to make sure they understand. Then it's up to them.

Patients sometimes ask me to manipulate the system for them. A common example is with disability. I have been appalled at the poor decisions that I have seen made by social security doctors who don't really know my patients and make life-changing decisions based upon partial information.

I have also seen patients try to get disability when they and I both know that they don't deserve it. At times like this, it is necessary that I be their doctor and not their best friend.

There are situations where I feel justified in challenging a system that inadequately protects my patients' rights. I am first and foremost my patients' defender. The current system of health care doesn't always do an adequate job of protecting and defending the rights of patients, and in certain situations, I will do what I legally can do to be my patients' advocate.

I feel that when I accept a patient into my practice, there is an implied contract to do everything within my power to help us work together. At times I feel that patients expect me to do it all myself. They then wonder why they don't get the desired outcome!

"Just a Little R. E. S. P. E. C. T."

Like Aretha Franklin and everyone else in the world, I want a little respect. It is not handed out freely to any of us. Rather, it needs to be earned through one's actions and hard work.

Anyone who has gone to school for twenty-five to thirty years deserves some respect, if nothing else, for tenacity and fortitude. You can't be a quitter and be a doctor; you earn that degree! Whether it's through hard work, stubbornness, or just sheer craziness isn't the issue.

It is disturbing to see a loss of respect for a person with a medical degree. Doctors are certainly not saints, but they are, for the most part, not the money-grubbing egotistical lot that many people perceive them to be.

Headlines in newspapers and on television sensationalize the things that bad doctors do, and they offer little to counterbalance this opinion. I can see the erosion of respect for doctors in patients' faces and in their attitudes. Trust has been damaged by the media and by the legal profession, but doctors have also done their part in allowing this to happen. They have been apathetic, unsympathetic, and sometimes downright greedy.

Managed care has turned the public into "doctor shoppers," but many people don't have a choice but to go where the winds of managed care blow them. One week they are with one company and one set of doctors; the next week they are with a different company and a totally different set of doctors. Managed care is the "free agency" of medicine, where there is little loyalty and people have the "show me the money" philosophy.

The result has been the erosion of the traditional bond between the doctor and his patient that was characterized by faith, trust, and loyalty. There are times when this special bond still exists, but it is rare and harder to find than before. I have seen it more commonly with my older patients who came from a generation of different values.

Doctors don't deserve respect if they are bad doctors or for having a lot of initials after their names. But give them the benefit of the doubt that they worked hard to get where they are to improve the quality of their patients' lives.

The Natural

I have been told from the time I was a teenager that I would make a good doctor because I had a "good bedside manner." No, I was never told that I looked like Robert Redford, darn it!

I guess people saw a soft-spoken young man with a tender heart and a caring nature and thought that I would be a "natural." I still receive that compliment, and I enjoy it immensely. However, having a "good bedside manner" is not at all natural for most of us, including me at times. It is something that can be improved upon and modified over the years. Each person has his or her own way of reaching out to others and needs to develop the techniques that work for him or her.

The most rewarding experiences that I have had as a doctor have been as a result of the bond that is formed with a patient that comes from a mutual goal being fulfilled. The things that I enjoy are found in a simple smile, a look in the eyes, or a touch of the hand.

Sometimes it is found in a hug or a note of appreciation. I have saved a collection of cards and notes from my patients that have touched my heart and my soul over the years. I will share some of them with you later. Other than the fulfillment of seeing a patient get well, the real enjoyment of being a doctor for me is found in my relationships with people and seeing how we affect each other's lives.

The things that I have found that people most appreciate are the time that I spend with them and the fact that I listen to them and try to understand them. The complaints that I most often hear about other doctors are: "So and so just doesn't take any time with me" or "He just won't listen to what I have to say."

One patient even told me about another doctor that would only take on one complaint per session. Usually, the doctors who are well liked are appreciated for the time they take with their patients and for their understanding and compassion.

Older people in particular are lonely and just need someone to talk to. A visit to a doctor's office is the major event of the day or even week for some of my patients. Doctors need to realize that the time and understanding given to these people is priceless.

My office staff pitches in and tries to make my office a comfortable place for people to visit. We can give them such incredible happiness by just taking time with them. Doctors are often guilty of thinking that their time is more important than anyone else's. Physicians need to remember that it is important to everyone. When the truth is told, older people probably have a lot less of it than we do.

I actually had one older patient ask me if I thought my time was more valuable than his. How do you answer a question like that? His response to my being late forced me to think about my response. My initial reaction was "yes," but after I thought about it for a while, I realized that we all have a limited time on this earth, and we all must make the most of it. Is my time really more valuable than another human being's because I'm a doctor?

Most people are the centers of their own universe, and patients commonly become frustrated when they have to wait to be seen by the physician or if they feel that their problems are being slighted.

I try my best to see patients on time and efficiently, but sometimes emergencies get in the way, or Murphy's Law makes me run late for my appointments. I try to have the attitude that my patients will understand if I tell them that I have to prioritize my time; they are no less important than anyone else. Ninety-nine per cent of the time, people don't disappoint me.

Fatigue and Burnout from an Overdose of Other People's Problems

---

"Said one psychiatrist to another: 'How do you handle sitting and listening to people's problems all day long?' Response: 'Who listens?'"

My interactions with my patients have led to many happy moments along with quite a few trials and tribulations. Often after a day of listening to an earful of problems, I come home worn out both mentally and physically. It consumes a lot of energy to listen to other people's problems day in and day out, assuming that you really listen.

No matter how fatigued this makes me, I can't afford to "run on empty." I owe it to my family to be able to help with issues around the house. I can't go home and say, "Sorry, but I gave at the office." That won't cut it! I owe it to my family members to have time and energy for them at the end of the day.

I periodically go through "burnout," and there are many times when I need to just get away from it all. Burnout may be the reason why some doctors rush in and out of patients' rooms and only appear to be hearing and not listening. I have seen some doctors walk in, examine a patient, and literally talk while they walk out the door. Sometimes they don't say anything at all, and the patient feels like he or she goes home empty handed.

What's the answer? Decreasing my time with patients is not a good compromise, and I would rather find ways to continue to listen without getting worn out and exhausted from the experience. I have had to find ways to revitalize my own energy levels when they have been drained.

I have also come to realize that I have my own limitations when it comes to dealing with people's problems; I can only tackle so many obstacles at one time and still be able to deal with the problems in my own life.

It has been essential to find ways to renew my spirit and keep enough energy for the important things. Personal renewal is essential not only for my patients' health but for mine as well. I can't take care of others if my own tank is empty! I'll discuss this more in a later section.

Intimacy and Physical Contact with Patients

"Sexual contact that occurs concurrent with the physician-patient relationship constitutes sexual misconduct."

Sect. 8., AMA Code of Medical Ethics

Temptation is always knocking on a doctor's door, and it takes a strong person to maintain strict boundaries when it comes to sex and intimacy, especially if you are in a room alone with an attractive patient. Doctors are human beings who happen to also be professionals. We are supposed to empathize and feel for our patients, yet we need to know when to inhibit our basic human instincts. Unfortunately, this isn't always easy, especially when patients are flirtatious and scantily clad, sometimes in sexy lingerie, often in nothing at all.

There is no immunity to the reaction of seeing a pleasing human body, and I have seen literally thousands of both beautiful and pretty gross sights over the years! The question is what to do about the natural chemical reaction that occurs when you see someone whom you are attracted to and you happen to also be her doctor. Where do you draw the line?

Not everyone agrees that doctors and patients should resist their attractions and abstain from physical and sexual contact. The AMA, and quite a few physicians and lawyers, vehemently disagree with the concept of doctor-patient intimacy. Let me explain why.

There are four main reasons why a code for sexual misconduct exists.

- Physical intimacy detracts from the goals of medicine, which are to help people with their illness, pain, and suffering. It clouds the picture and makes it hazy.
- A sexual relationship may exploit the vulnerability of the patient. As I have said before, patients are vulnerable, due to physical or psychological illness, to the comfort and caring that they receive from their doctor. The doctor's power over them could turn into exploitation. Fifty percent of "victims" have borderline personalities, which indicates psychiatric illness.[3] Others have chronic low self-esteem while many confuse "loving with caring."
- Intimacy may obscure the doctor's objectivity, and finally,
- Intimacy may be ultimately detrimental to the patient's well-being.

What does a doctor do if he feels that he needs intimacy with one of his patients?

"At a minimum, a physician's ethical duties include terminating the physician-patient relationship before initiating a dating, romantic, or sexual relationship with the patient."

AMA Code regarding Sexual Misconduct

The Texas Medical Practice Act states: "In the context of medical treatment, a sexual relationship with a patient is absolutely prohibited. Even if a termination of the professional relationship occurs, as long as there is a perceived relationship in the eyes of the patient...the physician is at risk for disciplinary action."[4] The key words here are "perceived relationship."

Doctors who are the most likely to be vulnerable to having physical relationships with their patients are usually frustrated with their medical practice and have trouble extracting satisfaction from their professional relationships with their patients. They also tend to have trouble with intimacy in their own personal relationships and have been found to have strong narcissistic qualities.

I have marveled at the fact that in a survey of sixteen hundred doctors, 3 percent admitted to having had sex with a patient, 4 percent to having dated a patient, while 20 percent knew other doctors who had dated or been intimate with their patients![5]

There is also the issue of "touching." As I have said before, I love to reach out and touch other human beings, but I have learned to be careful both about how I touch people and about whom I touch. Not everyone is receptive to being touched, even very innocently. Let me give you an example of problems that I have encountered from seemingly innocent patient contact.

I referred a patient to a doctor in a nearby community for a second opinion. The patient was very distraught after the visit and felt that the doctor had inappropriately touched her breast during the physical examination.

Cardiologists often feel a PMI, or Point of Maximal Impulse, below the breast. I am sure that the doctor had felt for the PMI but had not explained this to the patient. The patient didn't understand that the doctor was performing a normal examination. The doctor's problem was that he had not explained this to her. She was angry, and although she didn't file a report, she was left with a perception that was totally opposite from the physician's intention.

I have learned to explain the different parts of my examination to my patients because they can easily misinterpret what I am doing. It is easy for a doctor in a hurry to assume that patients understand the fine art of a physical exam.

Doctors make these false assumptions because they are fatigued and under pressure. It's an excellent idea to have a third party in the room so that there won't be a "your word against mine" type of situation that is often the result of a simple misunderstanding.

I still hug some of my patients, especially my eighty-year-olds. A lot of the elderly ones would think that I was upset with them if I didn't. The "hug" part of the visit is something that we both look forward to when they come to the office, and it sometimes means more to them than anything else that I say or do. As a matter of fact, it is often better medicine than any prescription that I could write.

All it takes is one accusation to ruin a reputation, a career, or a marriage. It's a pity that we can't entrust all of our patients with hugs! It is very difficult in this age of sexual exploitation and lawsuits to do some things that come naturally. A doctor must think about both his verbal and nonverbal communication and the impact that it has on his patients.

Doctors need to be very careful about enacting their fantasies concerning their patients. They belong only in dreams and in X-rated movies. It's not worth the risk for anyone involved!

Gifts and Symbols of Appreciation

Patients often want to show me their appreciation. My favorite items are the letters and cards that they have sent me that display their emotions and affection for me, as a doctor, and as someone special in their lives. I am going to show my favorites in a later section entitled, "Letters from the Heart."

Food comes in a close second with cookies and baked goods always finding a welcome mat at the front door. My office staff is often the object of this display of affection. Even when the cookies are meant for me, my staff has to be sure that they are good enough for me to eat!

Doctors need to be careful about the gifts that they allow themselves to receive from their patients. Other than food and letters, I start to get a little uneasy when my patients give me more expensive items, such as Mont Blanc pens, etc.

I look at the gift as not only a gift, but if it is extravagant or comes from a young person of the opposite sex, as also possibly having a motive behind it. It may be a symbol of affection, or it could be a conscious or subconscious effort to influence the way I take care of "the giver." There may be expectations behind it. It may indicate that "the giver" wants to pursue an intimate relationship, or it could be a subtle way to manipulate me into giving him or her special consideration, such as: "Doc, how about getting me in to see you earlier?" or "Can't you prescribe that pain medication for me? I don't have the time to go back to my other doctor?" If I accept an expensive gift, then it might send a message that I don't want to send, and it makes it hard to say "no" in the future to special requests.

If "the giver" is a young woman who is about my age or younger, I would be more concerned than if it came from an Arab sheikh whose custom was to give gifts to friends to show appreciation. There are cultural, age, and gender issues to consider when I decide whether to accept a gift. To the people of some cultures, my refusal might even be an insult.

As a rule, I love it when my patients show their respect and appreciation. I would be lying if I said that it didn't make me feel good deep inside. But I would rather have the cards and letters (and the cookies, of course) than anything else.

It's another boundary for the doctor to keep. But I have to admit that I sometimes wish that I had practiced medicine when doctors were paid in hens and clothes and didn't have to worry about Medicare and HMO's.

How Do You Say "No" to an Eighty-Year-Old?

"Doctor Farber, I have an 'erotic,' I mean, an 'erratic' heartbeat."

My Very Frisky Eighty-Year-Old Patient

It is hard to say "no" to an eighty-year-old, especially if she compliments you and tells you how sexy you look!

My patient caught me as I was passing in the hallway one day and told me to get "my sexy little ass" into the room. I did exactly what she asked! How could I refuse? She said that she enjoyed seeing her sexy doctor. I told her to come back as often as she wanted. Future visits were on the house!

I remember examining another eighty-year-old woman with an ophthalmoscope, an instrument used for eye examination. She commented halfway through the exam: "Doctor, that's the closest a man has been to me in years! Keep examining me for as long as you'd like. Just don't find anything wrong!"

Outwardly I blushed at these comments, but inside I smiled and was amused by the "reverse" sexual harassment. I also knew that they wouldn't sue me for joking right back with them.

My patients are living proof that although "there's snow on the roof, there's fire in the furnace." It's nice when you get to the age when you can say what you think and not worry about the consequences. Old age has its benefits!

Patient Portraits and Personalities

My experience has been that there are a number of different types of patient personalities. The complainers, shoppers, talkers, easy listeners, Doctor "Wannabes," procrastinators, frequent flyers, manipulators, and ramblers are some of the more common ones. I would like to paint a brief portrait of each one.

The Complainers or "Wolf-Criers"

There are chronic complainers whom I cannot make happy no matter what I do. They thrive on attention! I think that these people receive "secondary gain" from being ill because it brings the attention that they need from friends and loved ones. They just can't seem to ever get well.

In the meantime, they often gripe about their care, the office staff, or life in general. It is an interesting statistic that people who are dissatisfied with a doctor tell an average of twenty people, whereas satisfied patients share their experiences with only three. Somehow it doesn't seem fair.

Sometimes people are just depressed. Many of my complainers are just looking for someone to listen. Depression is an illness in itself and can be treated. A small dose of an antidepressant at times makes all the difference in the world and can turn a "complainer" into a "happy camper."

Complainers also are difficult to handle medically because they are the "wolf-criers." Sometimes it is hard to know when to take their complaints seriously because they complain and whine so much. They will then suddenly have a real medical problem when you least expect it. "The boy [or girl] who cried wolf" makes one of the most difficult patients for doctors to deal with. It's a challenge to maintain objectivity.

The Talkers

"If God had wanted us to talk more than listen, He would have given us two mouths instead of two ears."

Ken Blanchard, *We Are the Beloved*

The talkers usually come in carrying notes and lists of questions in their hands. Sometimes they have memorized a speech that they want to give the moment you walk in the room. Their most interesting characteristic is that they won't let me get a word in edgewise.

I often have wondered why they even bother coming to the doctor at all. I find myself thinking, "My God, won't they ever shut up?"

Talkers just don't have the patience to listen and tend to think that what they have to say is all-important. I usually have to interrupt them repeatedly just to ask a question, let alone say something important.

Sometimes it is not the patient who does the talking; sometimes the family won't let the patient get a word in edgewise. I often have to coax the relatives not to speak for their loved ones. Only the patient can tell me how he feels, that is, if he is allowed to!

Some people actually prefer that their spouses do the talking. For others, it is obviously embarrassing and irritating. It is nice to know that it irritates others besides me.

I'll ask: "What did your chest pain feel like?"

The spouse replies: "Well, he felt a sharp pain right in the middle of his chest, and it went to his back and down his arm and made him feel so terrible that **I just couldn't take it anymore**!"

Often people talk so that they don't have to listen. Doctors are as guilty of this as everyone else.

The Shoppers

Sometimes, I feel like shouting to my patients: "**Attention, Doctor Shoppers**!"

We live in a consumer-oriented and driven society. Now, more than ever, we shop for the best buys and have more money to spend than any other society in the world. We tend to look at things and people as "commodities." That unfortunately includes doctors.

We are probably the most spoiled society in the world, or it could be that we just have misguided priorities. Many people would rather spend money on cigarettes and alcohol than on their medical bills.

It is interesting that when some people are having a heart attack, they are grateful and incredibly thankful; yet after they have recovered, they neglect themselves and forget to see me in the office. They also somehow forget to pay their bills.

Fortunately, they don't make up the majority of my patients. They are usually the ones who need me again in the future. Then I hear all kinds of excuses, like "My gosh, has it been that long?" or "I really meant to pay that bill, but I've been so busy."

The true shoppers are those who are in the market for doctors who will tell them what they want to hear or who will give them a prescription for a pain pill or sedative. They usually go from one doctor to the next in search of a diagnosis that they feel fits their symptoms or in search of the "ultimate pill" that will solve their problems with the least amount of work on their part.

The hardest thing for some people to hear is that a doctor can't find anything wrong with them. People often need validation for their symptoms. They feel that there has to be something that has been missed if all the tests turn out normal. Some people just want an easy way out, one that is, of course, cheap, easy to take, and makes them feel good.

In my twenty years of medical experience, shoppers will eventually find what they are looking for. Some doctor somewhere will give them a diagnosis or perform a surgery that may not be necessary or give them a pain pill. They keep coming back for more, as long as the doctor gives them what they want.

We are taught that the American consumer is always right, even when he or she goes to the doctor. And there are plenty of doctors out there who are willing to take your money and allow you to consume even more. One good thing about managed care is that it has put some controls on how many doctors a patient can see. It has limited the patients' shopping spree and the doctors' spending spree.

The Easy Listeners

These are my favorite patients. They actually keep their appointments and listen to what I have to say! They ask questions but are willing to let me speak and to hear me out. Sometimes this description best fits the patient who has not gotten to know me well or feels safe communicating with me.

They sometimes then transform into talkers, but usually they are the more passive and compliant patients who follow instructions well. They are less challenging than some of the other types of personalities that I deal with, which is often a welcome relief at the end of a long day.

Usually patients don't fit neatly into this or any other particular category. There is a lot of overlap, and people often change from one to another depending upon what is going on in their lives and how secure they feel in our relationship.

The Doctor "Wannabes"

I have cared for quite a few patients who are "frustrated doctors." They should have gone to medical school, and they usually act like they have medical degrees. No matter what I say, they know what's best. They tend to be on the obsessive-compulsive side, a lot like doctors, and are usually the ones that are up at all hours checking their blood pressures or pulse rates. What's worse is that they call me at all hours wondering why they have insomnia!

There are some patients who know their bodies better than any doctor ever could. Diabetics, in particular, know their response to insulin and how to treat their diabetes better than most doctors who care for them.

I usually allow them to treat themselves unless they run into trouble because I know that they understand their bodies better than I do. I have seen doctors ignore patients who claim to know how their bodies will react to a situation or a medication. The results are usually not pretty for the patient or for the doctor.

The remaining "wannabes" are responsible for a lot of my sleepless nights. Very often they wonder why things are not going well in spite of the fact that they have adjusted their own medications!

They are also responsible for a lot of my gray hairs. I usually need a soundproofed padded room to ventilate my frustrations after I have finished trying to convince them to let me be the doctor. "Too many cooks spoil the broth."

The Procrastinators

These patients are hard to understand, and the only way that I can rationalize what they do is that they must have an awful lot of denial that they are anything but healthy.

My experience has been that they are predominantly male and often middle-aged. I find it interesting that they usually call me on a Saturday night or go to the E.R. on a weekend after having had symptoms for days or often weeks.

They are like babies and want to be delivered at inopportune times. I can't hold back the inevitable question: "Why in the world did you wait so long?" Usually the response is that they didn't think it was anything serious. Denial is a powerful defense mechanism and has killed many of my patients.

I remember one young forty-five-year-old man who came to the hospital with an acute myocardial infarction, or heart attack. One big problem is that he had refused to believe that he had been having cardiac symptoms for weeks. He even refused to believe that he was having a heart attack even when we told him that his EKG was definitive in the E.R.

It took an hour of convincing to finally make him realize that we had to do an emergency catheterization. Time is crucial in this setting, and I was becoming frustrated. Finally his wife and the E.R. nurse convinced him of the critical nature of the situation. He received the care he needed and eventually did well.

There are others whom I have cared for who have been less fortunate. I remember numerous patients over the course of my medical career that delayed necessary medical care because something else in their lives had to be taken care of that was more important. Sometimes they had to get their affairs in order, but very often patients delay their care for relatively minor reasons. I have heard people cancel doctor's visits because of hair appointments. Sometimes they even say they are too sick to go to the doctor!!!

Two or three of them didn't make it to the next appointment with me. They kept their appointment with God instead. There's an old saying that is so true: "You can lead a horse to water, but you can't make him drink."

Whoever thought of this saying must have known many a doctor's patients.

The Frequent Flyers

These patients generally require tender loving care. Sometimes they are lonely and oftentimes the visit to my office is a bright spot in their week. They know that I care, and visiting me is akin to visiting a friend or a relative. Many of my older patients tell me I am like a son to them. I am often younger than some of their children, so the comparison is not that far-fetched.

I call them "frequent flyers" because they are in my office a lot. They are very pleasant to deal with and generally listen to what I have to say. Sometimes I feel like my office is a home away from home for them.

When I was an intern and resident at Ben Taub and the VA hospital, we had certain patients who routinely came to the E.R. at Thanksgiving and Christmas. Their health was no worse than usual at these times, but they were lonely, had no family, and literally had nowhere else to go.

We often found "reasons" to put them in the hospital because we knew that there they could find a warm bed, something to eat (they actually appreciated hospital food), and companionship. At that time, we made adjustments in the system to accommodate their needs, and I have no regrets.

If I could do the same thing today, I would. The new world of medicine is not that compassionate.

The Manipulators

This is an important subgroup of the other personality types but is so common that it deserves some discussion. "Control" is the basic element of the manipulator. There are a lot of "control freaks" out there, and most of them don't wear white coats. This could turn into a real power struggle and a tug of war between doctor and patient.

It is important to remember that for every manipulator to be successful, there has to be someone who allows himself or herself to be manipulated, either consciously or on a subconscious level. There is often a fight for control between patient and doctor. The struggle may be over medications—patients often demanding controlled substances such as narcotic pain medications—or it may be a result of patients trying to "play doctor." Like I said in the previous section, one doctor is enough in a doctor-patient relationship. Two gets kind of crowded.

It is not uncommon for adults to throw temper tantrums when they don't get their way. This is often true when patients threaten to find another doctor or sue me if they don't get what they want. I usually "call their bluff" and give them their records on the spot: "Don't waste my time anymore; go find someone else to give you want you want!"

The problem is that there are too many doctors waiting with prescription pads who have no problem writing prescriptions for Valium or Vicodin. Patients who doctor-shop often find what they are looking for if they are persistent.

It is so sad to see doctors give in to this kind of pressure. I think some are afraid of losing their patients and are insecure. Unfortunately, there are too many who are just downright greedy and give patients what they want because of money. Some probably just don't care or want to avoid conflict. Others may have just given up fighting and just want to take the easy way out.

The Ramblers

The ramblers keep me focused. When I ask them where their pain is located, the response is something like, "Pain, well, let me tell you about pain; my grandmother used to have sciatica, and, boy, that was no fun at all."

With ramblers, I have to constantly use my energy to herd them back in the direction that will take us where we need to go. I need specific answers to very specific questions, and it's not that I don't want to hear about grandma's sciatica but that I need to get other important information first. Then we can socialize if there is time.

The ramblers are interesting because they at times seem to intentionally avoid the subject. This could be a form of denial. Dealing with them is like trying to herd a bunch of cats, or doctors, for that matter.

Looking at the Bright Side

The bright side is that I get a lot more out of my positive interactions with the majority of my patients than I lose in emotional and mental energy. I feel needed and appreciated, and I have known no better "high" than knowing that someone's life has been changed for the better by my efforts. I have come to realize that I affect people's lives in a lot more ways as a doctor than I had originally thought. Let me give you an example of a little old man whom I will never forget, and who gave me an important gift.

I took care of an elderly man who was near the end of his life with both a bad heart and bad lungs. He knew he was near death and that his time was short. He was trying to have his family near him as much as possible before his time came, and he was trying to reconcile with an estranged son whom he had not seen in a year and a half.

During a visit to his bedside one morning, he started to tell me that his son had refused to come visit him, even as he lay near death. He was near tears as he recounted his efforts to try to communicate to his son that he was sincere in his desire for reconciliation. I listened and did not know what to say, so I just continued to listen.

He told me he had prayed and asked his son for forgiveness, and it was obvious that he needed to make peace with his son before he died. I didn't know how to help him, so I tried to say something comforting. I sounded less than profound; the right words just wouldn't come to me. I couldn't do much but keep him physically comfortable until his time came because I didn't know how to comfort him spiritually.

At the end of our conversation, he told me something that I will never forget. He said that every minute of my visits with him made him happy and that he looked forward to talking to me again. He grabbed my hand and just held it. He and I both had tears in our eyes as I left the room.

I knew that there was no better medicine that I could give him than just being there for him, and I knew that there was no better medicine for my heart and soul than what I had just experienced. This man had given me an important gift, one that helped me as much as anything that I had experienced in life. He gave me enlightenment and tranquility in exchange for sitting by him and holding his hand.

By the way, he and his son reconciled a week after our conversation. He eventually did go home to spend his last days with his family, with the peace that he was so desperately seeking.

Sometimes "just being there" is enough; little or nothing needs to be said. A lot can be conveyed by non-verbal communication, and this is sometimes the best kind. When patients have faith in me, they often want me at their bedside even when I am not the one performing the surgery.

I have come to realize that it was for moments like these that I became a doctor. All the fatigue, frustration, and difficult times in training and the long hours in the daily grind of my practice were worth these precious moments, even if they were heart breaking.

I could never have felt the same satisfaction from doing anything else, and my soul is the richer for it. I have realized that I don't have to see large numbers of patients or make large amounts of money to feel successful. One patient like this is all it takes. Quantity is less important than quality.

This man made me understand that patients truly do have a gift to give that is as great as any in creation, as long as we open our eyes to it. By their living examples, they can teach us how to both live and die with dignity. The old man showed me both.

Allowing Patients to Be Proactive Teachers

I encourage my patients to be proactive in their care. I want them to take an active role in something that is so personal and vitally important as their health. This makes me work even harder and keeps me on my toes.

I realize that my patients are sometimes going to disagree with my recommendations, but I don't try to arm-twist them into submission. Most of them are adults and have a right to make up their own minds. Coercion is not in my game plan.

My goal is to present them with the facts and my best recommendations, even if it involves seeing another specialist to get a second opinion. From that point on, it is **their** decision and **their** choice. Sometimes it is not easy to bite my tongue when I think they are making a mistake. But I try to remember my place: I am their doctor, not their keeper.

Patients are educating themselves by reading journals and scouring the Internet for information about how to treat their problems. I have learned almost as much from talking to my patients as I have from reading the major medical journals. One patient introduced me to *The Harvard Heart Letter*. I have found it a delight to read, and it keeps me informed about subjects that are of interest to my patients. I refer to it often when I talk with my patients, and I now subscribe to it myself.

Doctors need to bridge the "information gap" with their patients and realize that the best answers are not always in their own journals:

"In February, *The New England Journal of Medicine* made headlines for its acknowledgment that some authors of a series on drug therapy had received major research support through their institutions from pertinent companies or were consultants for these companies at the time they were asked to write the articles."[6]

This was an obvious conflict of interest found in a well-respected medical journal and should make physicians realize that they may not always have "perfect" information. Patients look to their doctors for information and solid medical advice. It is crucial that they stay current with the latest literature, keeping an open mind to things that are not in the time-honored journals that they have read for decades. A lot of times, patients bring good solid information to the table.

"Failure to recognize and bridge an information gap with our patients makes the relationship vulnerable to conflict and controversy....As physicians, it is our responsibility to become more savvy—about the media and public information, about our patients and their perspectives, and about medicine overall....At the same time, we are

well served to recognize our personal limitations and to understand the boundaries of our abilities."[7]

Earlier in my career, I would have felt threatened by the idea that patients could be my teachers. I was supposed to be the expert; that's why I went to school for all those years, and that's what people expect me to be. I have learned, however, that my patients can teach me not only about medicine but also about many of life's lessons.

A lot of my patients are senior citizens and have a lot of experience with life. Many have tried to teach me some of what they have learned and to give me advice. There are important take-home messages in many of my daily interactions. My life has been enriched by the knowledge that my patients have passed on to me. I owe them a debt of gratitude for that.

A common saying among doctors is that general practitioners know "a little about a lot" of things whereas specialists know "a lot about very little." Over time, I have come to realize that you can't know everything about anything. It's just that it took me years to admit it to myself and to my patients.

I feel that I became a better doctor when I stopped being insecure. In the very beginning, I was afraid that I would not know how to relate to my patients. I was even worried they wouldn't like me enough to keep coming to me as their doctor. I have developed self-confidence as time has passed, and I no longer worry about maintaining a façade. What my patients see is what they get. I try to just be myself and relate to them on a personal but professional level.

Skepticism—Healthy or Dangerous?

A corollary of living in an age of communication and of being a litigious society is that everyone has heard or read horror stories about the care that someone else has received. Most often these stories are blown out of proportion by relatives or friends, but they generally have the effect of causing skepticism and mistrust of physicians.

So many of my patients have heard about the terrible complications that have happened to others during routine procedures. I respond by trying to give reassurance, which is difficult in some situations because a lot of people have already made their minds up about what they are going to do before coming to the doctor's office.

Living in this state of skepticism makes my job more difficult, but I realize that it is usually healthy if people can keep an open mind. In today's world, people tend to mistrust doctors. It is harder to find loyalty than it was years ago, but sometimes loyalty can be blind and trust, misplaced. Doctors need to prove themselves more than ever in today's world.

Skepticism has both a healthy side and an unhealthy side to it. I want my patients to believe in me but to also be proactive and check out alternatives on their own. Sometimes it is hard to find the right balance between loyalty and healthy skepticism.

Unfortunately, both negative publicity and negative reporting by the media have raised anxiety and concern about medical care. People want to know who their doctor is now more than ever. They want to know the person that they are placing their trust in. Having a medical degree isn't enough these days. And it probably shouldn't be.

To Be a Friend or Not to Befriend?

Whether or not a patient likes me is really not all that important, although I can't see people wanting me to be their doctor if they didn't like me as a human being. Friendship, in fact, sometimes makes my job tougher. To maintain my credibility and effectiveness with patients, I often need to be painfully blunt and even parentally stern. Friendship sometimes makes it harder to say the difficult words that need to be said.

No matter how hard I try to not become emotionally involved with my patients, emotional ties are hard to avoid, especially if I've known the patient for a long time. Friendship and sensitivity make it easier to empathize with people, but they also force you to feel the pain of others and sometimes lose your objectivity.

I have learned to live with the downside of my sensitive nature and realize that I am who I am, and I couldn't change even if I wanted to. I feel that my patients are better off because I am caring and sensitive to their needs.

Patients want to like their doctors and generally want to be liked in return. That is human nature. It is an honor to be considered a friend by many of my patients, but my job is not necessarily to befriend them. Very few of my patients are what I would consider to be close friends, but I care about all of them as unique individuals with special needs.

I'll show you later how my relationships with my patients have benefited me both as a private individual and as a doctor when I talk about one of my favorite patients named Cramer.

Can a Person Have Too Much Faith in His or Her Doctor?

I want my patients to be loyal and faithful. Their belief in me helps me immeasurably in my ability to help them. But the faith that can heal a patient can also be dangerous when it interferes with his or her ability to get good medical care.

I would like to share with you a situation that demonstrates that having extreme faith in a doctor can be counterproductive to a patient's well-being. It involves a woman who had been under my care for years. While I was on vacation, she became ill and needed a heart catheterization. She refused to let the doctor on call for me perform the procedure, and she suffered a heart attack and died before I returned home.

Her faith in me had actually led to her untimely death, and she died because she couldn't trust someone else fully. I felt sad and guilty when I found out what had happened. My desire and struggle to have my patients believe in me had actually worked against one of them!

Sometimes patients have so much faith in their doctor that they feel he can't make any mistakes. It seems that, in their eyes, he is almost superhuman. I am not sure which is worse, the "blind believer" or the annoying skeptic.

Check out your doctor as much as possible with your friends and local medical association. Find out if he has any history of drug-related problems or even felonies. Sometimes these problems are kept confidential, but you want to make sure you are putting your faith in someone who deserves it.

When a Patient Utters the "S" Word

There are times when a doctor-patient divorce is beneficial and necessary for everyone involved. Sometimes a patient might "fire" me, but I have regrettably been forced to terminate my relationship with some patients or at the very least to discourage certain patients from coming back to see me as their doctor. Let me tell you some of the reasons why:

- If the patient utters the "S—T" word, it is grounds for immediate action on my part. Shame on them! You know what I mean; I am talking about "suits," as in lawsuits. If patients sound litigious or even mention the word in my presence, they need to find another doctor. After years of trying to help people, I won't allow myself to be threatened or harassed by people who want to bully me into submission by threatening to sue me. This really pushes my "anger" button! A little voice in the back of my head yells: **Eject! Eject!**

- Dishonesty makes it difficult to give good medical care and leads to mistrust. Dishonesty can take many forms, some of which are grounds for immediately terminating the relationship. Some patients have gone so far as to change the number of pills on prescriptions that I have written for pain pills or sedatives. I have had no recourse but to fire patients for altering prescriptions and report them to the authorities. Sometimes, patients want me to manipulate the system by making them "disabled" when they really are not. It is really not all that difficult to emotionally detach yourself from the patients who want to abuse and cheat the system or from those who abuse my trust.
- If a patient is rude and ugly repeatedly to my staff or to myself, it makes it difficult to continue to provide good care. Everyone has the capacity to get rude under the right circumstances, and at times emotional outbursts are due to the stresses of being ill. Everyone has "bad hair days." Unfortunately, there are people who make a habit out of rudeness, and that is something that I just won't tolerate. It provides a negative environment both for me and for my staff and makes it less likely that I can effectively provide unbiased medical care for the patient.
- I have fired patients who have jeopardized their care through repeated noncompliance with any legitimate medical treatment. Some people just have a death wish, and I don't want to have any part of it. Sometimes they even bring me down emotionally with them in the process and drain my energy levels. They take my time away from people who want to help themselves.
- There are times when I am just mentally exhausted with an emotionally trying case. In these situations, I have recommended that my patients seek another opinion and a fresh look from an objective party. This is really

> not firing a patient but referring them elsewhere for their care when I feel that I have done all that I can do.

I don't relish the thought of firing patients, but sometimes it is in their best interests, as well as mine, for them to seek care elsewhere. Medicolegally, a doctor has to give proper notice to his patients and be careful not to abandon them without giving them ample time to find another healthcare provider.

I owe it to my patients to be honest with them when I feel that I can no longer function effectively as their physician.

One Patient's Response to Managed Care

The very heart and soul of medicine is at risk with the shifting of the winds of managed care. Let me give an example of a patient who would not permit himself to be manipulated by the system or be traded to the lowest bidder.

I had taken care of Ed for years before he was admitted to the hospital with chest pain. I had performed heart catheterizations on him in the past and knew his family almost as well as I knew him. Soon after Ed's admission, I performed a heart catheterization and found that he had developed a new blockage that was threatening to cause a heart attack.

I recommended a coronary angioplasty, which involves opening up the blocked artery with a balloon. He agreed to it after the options were discussed.

A day after the catheterization, I received a call from a case worker at the hospital who told me that someone had made a mistake in the front office and that I could no longer take care of Ed. His managed-care company had contracted with another medical group in the area. A phone call confirming this followed. The doctor reaffirmed the insurance company's position, and he went on to state that if the patient continued to be under my care, Ed would be totally responsible for his own hospital bills.

I reluctantly went to Ed to discuss this matter. I was frustrated, and I was afraid that this news might cause him to have a heart attack before his heart could be fixed. I was also angry with a managed-care coordinator who interrupted the care of my patient at a critical time, right in the middle of a hospitalization for a life-threatening problem. I saw the cold side of medicine in all its modern splendor.

To my surprise, Ed told me that he would personally pay for the remainder of his hospital stay and that he didn't want another doctor to perform the operation. He felt that his faith in me outweighed all other factors. I followed his wishes and performed the angioplasty, and he was forced to pay for it himself. The bill, not surprisingly, was rather large.

This is an example that is almost unheard of in the world of managed care. It makes me feel good inside to know a man whose faith could not be bought. He would not allow a cruel and insensitive system to beat him. I know that all of my patients could not have afforded to do this, but I felt honored that Ed placed this kind of faith in me.

More Typical Scenarios

It is not uncommon for me to admit a patient to the hospital who belongs to an HMO or PPO of which I am not a contracted member. Sometimes the hospital isn't contracted with the health plan either. These patients are often in life-threatening situations that require care to be delivered first and questions about insurance to be asked later. They are rightfully taken to the closest facility.

I spend hours taking care of patients in acute distress, performing life-saving procedures, and getting to know both them and their families. When they are stable, I am often forced by managed care to transfer these patients to the "participating" doctor and hospital, often forty-five minutes to an hour away.

The process involved usually requires multiple frustrating phone calls, often taking hours of my time. The frustrations mount as I am put on hold or have problems finding out just who to talk to. Often the right hand doesn't know what the left is doing!

Perhaps the most frustrating thing for me, and often for my patients, is not the unnecessary time consumption, but the fact that our system threatens to extinguish the relationship that we have worked hard to build. It is extremely frustrating to have established a rapport with a patient and then be forced to send them elsewhere. It is even more frustrating to know that I could have done the same or a better job than the doctor that I sent them to.

It is just as embarrassing to go into a patient's room to tell him or her that it would be to his or her benefit to stay in the hospital one more day only to have the insurance company decide that the extra day is medically "unnecessary."

Calling the insurance company to validate the need for the extra day and documenting the facts on the chart is essential. It's very frustrating to explain medical necessity to someone who sits at a desk somewhere hundreds or thousands of miles away and doesn't know my patients or their needs.

Managed care does not provide a good climate for my relationships with my patients to thrive and prosper. Our system is a trust-destroyer and undermines a doctor's credibility with his patients. At times it is downright dangerous for the patient and increases the risks of being sued. Doctors and hospitals are held accountable for these important decisions and sometimes are hung out to dry by the managed care industry.

Every Doctor Needs a "Cramer"

Let me tell you about a patient who is the epitome of what makes the doctor-patient relationship special.

I took care of an ex-coal miner with "black lungs" seventeen years ago when I first went into practice. He died after a prolonged illness. The wife's name was Alberta, and we bonded almost immediately, partly because she's a "Yankee" just like me but mostly because she appreciated the concern that I had shown her husband.

Alberta is a descendent of German immigrants and is a woman of many virtues, one of the most obvious being loyalty. Her loyalty to her husband was evident during his illness, and she has become loyal to me over the years since her husband passed away.

My visits with "Cramer," as she likes to be called, are usually half social and half medically oriented. She asks me about how my life is going and is concerned with my happiness. She tells me about her life, often discusses her fears and her loneliness, and confides her innermost feelings. We eventually discuss her medical problems during her visits, but usually we first discuss how our lives our going.

I am board certified in both internal medicine and cardiology but only practice the latter. I am not hesitant to tell my patients that I am strictly a cardiologist. This doesn't sit well with Cramer because I am the only doctor she trusts. She has not developed faith in anyone else, and she has been upfront and told me that she wants me to take care of all of her medical problems.

This has posed an interesting dilemma for me because I have been very strict about my rule of not practicing internal medicine. With Cramer, I have allowed myself to make a little bit of a compromise. In her case, I go as far as I can within my comfort zone but generally advise her to see a specialist for most of her problems that I don't feel that I am capable of taking care of. The most important thing is that she has faith in my advice and in my recommendations. She just wants to talk to me about her problems and listens to what I have to say. She has that much faith in me.

I am touched by her love and faith. She considers herself my second mother and tells everyone that I am like a son to her. It's not a manipulation; she is obvious in her sincerity. She feels that she is family to both me and to my office staff. I believe that her visits to me are as important as are her visits to her family. And I have come to feel that her visits are important to me too because they remind me of why I am working hard at what I am doing.

She is a good example of the importance of having faith in your doctor. To give an example, Alberta called me at home one evening because she was upset and worried about not having been able to go to the bathroom for five days. I gave her advice about how to remedy the problem with medications and told her that she may have to go to the emergency room if things didn't improve.

Ten minutes later, she called me back and told me that after hearing my voice, she suddenly became able to move her bowels. I knew that I had a gift for healing but didn't realize that the sound of my voice had therapeutic (and even a cathartic) value. God is still making me aware of the talents that he has given me.

I have taken a lot of good-natured kidding since then, but it shows how important faith is in the healing of patients. Medicine may be better delivered with the sound of a voice and the touch of a hand than with all the expensive drugs in the world.

Cramer exemplifies the faith and loyalty that all doctors would love to have from their patients. I am proud to call her my patient and my friend. She is also an example of how being a doctor can be both challenging and rewarding at the same time. I would take one Cramer over a thousand less loyal and faithful patients.

There is a saying that there is "no doctor like a true friend." There is also no question that my ability to help Alberta is enhanced by our friendship and that the special nature of our relationship increases her faith.

In today's world of managed care, she represents a breed that is quickly becoming extinct. Her loyalty is becoming increasingly hard to come by. Maybe her age dictates a different set of values that sets her apart in the world of modern-day medicine. She represents old-fashioned virtues that I admire greatly. If people were to ask me later in life if I was happy that I had been a doctor, my response would be that what made it worthwhile were people like Cramer.

There is a definite risk that our rules and regulations may allow her values to become relics of history. What a shame it would be to sell her soul to the highest bidder and lose our own souls in the process.

They Can Make You or Break You!

Who are they? Patients, bankers, lawyers, insurance companies, and the government all affect the ebb and flow of my medical practice, but few have the ability to help or hurt me as much as my office staff. I can be the best doctor in the world, but if my office staff doesn't do its job well or is not professional, then my patients will find other doctors to treat them. Conversely, I could be the worst doctor in the world, and if I had caring, sensitive office people working with me, my patients would keep coming back for more.

My office staff is an extension of me. Everything that my staff members do reflects on me. What they tell me affects how I feel about a patient, and the reverse is true as well. My patients will respect me if my staff responds to them caringly, courteously, and professionally.

At times, and I am sure you are surprised to hear this, my patients must wait their turn to see me, sometimes longer than I would like. Good office personnel will talk to them, make them comfortable, and do what it takes to make them happy and feel good in moments of aggravation.

On the other hand, it is frustrating to hear from patients that their calls went unanswered, or that they were subjected to rudeness on the phone or at the office. This makes me cringe because it is not my style. But it is interpreted as being my style if those around me adopt that behavior. What's even worse is that people think that I condone and sanction it.

I have come to realize that my staff is my right arm, and sometimes my left. The staff members extend my ability to heal my patient, and they help me to go beyond the limits that fatigue and time impose. They are there listening when I am busy or in surgery or when I just can't do one more thing. They make my patients feel wanted rather than brushed off.

It took years for me to assemble a trustworthy, compassionate, hard-working office staff. What I look for in my staff is loyalty, trustworthiness, dedication, and compassion for my patients. When you find staff members like that, keep them and cherish them!

Role Models

When I was growing up, I read a book about the art of medicine. I followed the headlines about Denton Cooley and Michael DeBakey and all of the things that they were accomplishing in revolutionizing medicine. Christiaan Barnard was doing the first heart transplant in Capetown, South Africa, and I was watching *Star Trek* on television and saw "Bones" use his tricorder to diagnose his crew's problems in a futuristic view of medicine.

I was fascinated by what I read and saw, and it intrigued me enough to want to become part of this world. When I look back, these real and fictional characters helped to shape the kind of doctor that I wanted to be. I liked the idea of affecting people's lives for the better, but I was also determined to figure out what made these people tick.

I have been fortunate enough to meet two of these people. I would love to have been able to meet "Bones" in the future because I loved the way he would call himself an old country doctor no matter how much the future tried to change him. I still admire him when I watch the reruns, and I say to myself, "This is the kind of doctor that I want to be." He never sacrificed his values. No matter how much he used his tricorder, he still talked to Captain Kirk and to Spock as a country doctor would talk to his patients.

I met Denton Cooley as a cardiology fellow and was amazed to see his humanitarian side. A lot of people would hide behind their fame but not Dr. Cooley. He took the time to personally call me about the patients that I sent to him; but more importantly, I saw him take the time to go out to the waiting room to talk to each individual family of each patient that he operated on.

Considering he would routinely operate on twenty or thirty patients daily, that took considerable time out of his schedule. I was amazed to see him do this personally and not send one of his young trainees. To this day, I have admired him as much for his caring attitude as for any of his medical achievements. He doesn't distance himself from people because he is famous.

One of my most satisfying days as a doctor came when Dr. Cooley complimented me on my work. I have always admired Dr. Cooley, and earlier in this book, I compared him to another boyhood idol, calling him the "Mickey Mantle of Medicine." He hit a homerun with this fan when I saw him in action. His fame has obviously not prohibited him from showing that he is truly in touch with people's feelings.

Michael DeBakey has always been an enigma to me. I have never been able to talk to him privately, so I really can't say that I know or understand the man. I saw one side of him on rounds, and he was a man of few words. But whenever he said something, you listened!

He was all business in front of his colleagues, and I never saw any other side. He had a reputation for strictness, kind of like the old-fashioned schoolteacher. His values were to put the patient first, and he worked as hard as any doctor that I have ever seen.

I saw Dr. DeBakey at the hospital at all hours of the day and night. He is a man of abundant energy, a non-stop personality who takes a deep and sincere interest in his patients. I have referred to him as the "Lou Gehrig or Iron-Horse of Medicine" because of his longevity and dedication to hard work.

Fame did not keep him away from his patients, and I think that it probably made him work even harder. I wish that I could have gotten to know the man better, to see what makes him tick. As a teacher, there is no one who strives harder for perfection, and it is obvious that he works hard to maintain the traditions of medicine. I have never met anyone who could quite compare to him, and I doubt that there ever will be.

I have had two other role models who have taught me a lot about how to treat patients as people instead of as diseases or as things that needed fixing. They are both primary-care doctors who work alongside me in the small community of Conroe, Texas. Dr. Burrell Powell and Dr. Unal Gurol have both been in practice for thirty to forty years.

They know the history of medicine and their importance in the scheme of things. They embody old-fashioned values and ethics and take the time to talk to people. They know when to ask for help and when to put the welfare of their patients first. They still make house calls to patients on a routine basis, which is not common in the new world of medicine.

What I admire the most about them, however, are the values that they represent. Like my patient Cramer, they embody timeless ideals that we cannot allow to be buried by the winds of change. We must strive to help produce doctors who are more like them and preserve their legacies.

We can take the best of what the future of medicine has to offer and still be the "country doctors" of the past. Others have shown us the way. We need to recognize how important it is to follow the trail that they have blazed and not let the pressures of lawyers and politicians corrupt our ideals and values.

I want to be remembered as a doctor who was compassionate with his patients, stood by his ideals, and was not afraid to show that he was "human."

Let's not allow "Big Brother" to become a fulfilled prophecy. We need to keep the best of the past along with whatever we do in the present and future. Changes are necessary, but we cannot forsake the ideals and values that are at the heart of our profession.

Memories and Mementos from My Patients

My favorite memories and mementos from my patients are their hugs, best wishes, and prayers. Nothing material could match these tokens of appreciation. They have made everything that I have done more than worthwhile. They have touched my life and have profoundly affected me. I have saved several over the years that have meant a lot to me. I would like to share some of these with you.

Letters from the Heart

I want you to read several letters that exemplify how my patients have helped make my life richer. The purpose of printing selections of these letters is not for self-aggrandizement but to illustrate the profound effect that a doctor can have on his patients and vice-versa.

12-19-84

Dear Dr. Farber,

I just wanted to write you to let you know that my mom passed away Friday nite....She had made me promise to take her to see you on Jan 1st. I didn't think she had an appt. But I found one in her Bible. I just really wanted to tell you thank you—that I believe Moma really trusted you and held a special place in her heart for you. I believe you know that I but I wanted to tell you and also that I appreciate your human concern and taking time to talk to us. I think you are a good doctor and person....

Thanks and love....H and B

Wed. 29th, 1985

My Dear Dr. Farber,

Please forgive me for not writing to thank you for all you did to help keep Thad for us. Knowing you as a person and a doctor it was a difficult situation for you as well as it was us. That makes you very special to this family. I am trying to get on with my life, but its not easy. We had a good life together. In the twilight years of our lives is the time we all need someone more and we had that and you helped both of us to have more of them. Young people like yourself also need someone. I pray you will always have the things you want and need if you don't work your life away before. Take an 'ole woman's advice. Take some time out to relax, enjoy life some day you will find that it will be a lot easier on you.

The rest of my time will be spent on enjoying my family, keeping as well as possible and remembering the happy days Thad and I had, especially when all the pain has been tucked away. Again I thank you and all of your staff for the kindness and thoughts when needed most. Stay happy, well, and that will better your life.

Sincerely, B

Jan. 14, 1985

Dear Dr. Farber:

I wanted to take this moment to personally thank you for everything you did for me. It's quite obvious that without your help and ability to control the situation, I might now be a memory to dear friends and family.

Your concern and sensitivity to the situation represents the very best in your profession. Thank you again and I hope your success in life is worthy of what you deserve.

Regards, JS.

Dr. Farber,

Words can never express my appreciation about how much you cared about Robert. He loved all of you dearly and will watch over you all forever. Dr. Farber—you were his hero and I will always be grateful for your caring.

I will never forget any of you, Lovingly, S.B.

December 1, 1997

Dearest Steve,

This is an attempt to thank you for the care you gave to Clint. There are not enough words to cover what's in my heart.

I want you to know you accomplished what you told him you wanted to do with the infusions. You freed him from the repeated struggles for breath.

He died a very gently death and this was the answer to my most fervent prayer—and he got to die at home with us where he wanted to be.

We love you very much. R.B.

Dear Dr. Farber,

I want to thank you and your staff—Valerie, Charlene, Janet for being so kind to me.

There is no way I can repay your kindness, but I do thank you from the bottom of my heart. Without your help I could never make it financially. My prayers are out to all of you every day.

My love, A.C.

March 6, 2000

Dear Dr. Farber:

I just wanted to take a moment to let you know how much I appreciate you and your staff for all you did for me over the last 8 years. I know this is "just your job," but the way you treated me, both medically and personally, was unusually high caliber. Your "bedside manner" is superior to so many of the doctors I know. I always felt you were working hard for me and had my best interests in mind. I always felt better mentally after our appointments because of the serious manner in which you treated my atrial fib. I know that there are conditions a lot more serious than mine, but you gave me your undivided attention in every conference and never let me feel that you were in a hurry to just do something to get me out of the office.

Dr. Farber, I also was much impressed by the fact that you took the treatment of my condition to a certain point and were willing to refer me to another specialist when you felt you had done all you could for me.

Sincerely, R.M.

And one more:

Dear Steve and Staff:

When I saw this card, it reminded me of the feeling Paul and I have when we come into the office or call. It is a loving, caring kindness, something our world seems to have forgotten. Steve, you are like our own son. Paul and I lift you up in prayer each night. You are so special because God made you that way. He gave each of you the ability to make sad times, glad times.

We love you all. Paul and Euline

These are a few of my favorites from the samples of letters and cards that I have received over the years. These expressions of love and appreciation give me a renewed sense of purpose when I am tired and frustrated. They make it all worthwhile, especially when I feel like nothing is going right.

Looking back, it is interesting that my patients had tried to look out for my interests and welfare almost as much as I have theirs. I wish that I had heeded their advice at times. I regret not having listened to the wisdom that comes only with age and experience. My patients have been wiser about life than their doctor. At times, they have been the teachers, and I have been their pupil.

I would like to express my feelings and appreciation to my patients. What they have taught me over the years has left a powerful and lasting impression on my being. They have taught me how to laugh, how to cry, how to live, and, yes, how to die.

A Story of Life and Death

I am going to preface the next chapter by relating two experiences with patients that have taught me a lot about death. Mr. Z. was a middle-aged male and, unfortunately, had suffered what is referred to as sudden death or cardiopulmonary arrest in the field. Attempts at resuscitation were successful but only after the patient had been exposed to prolonged hypoxia or lack of oxygen.

Mr. Z. never woke from his coma. The neurologists felt that he had minimal brain wave activity and that he would remain in a vegetative state permanently. All of the physicians on the case, including myself, felt that the situation was terminal and that if life support was removed, Mr. Z. would not be able to survive more than a few minutes or hours at the most.

We had a meeting with the family, and after expressing our opinions about Mr. Z.'s condition, they expressed their desire to terminate life support. They were evoking a living will that the patient had declared before his heart attack.

There was much prayer, and I prayed with them over their difficult decision. The decision was not easy for me as their physician. They said their goodbyes. And then something interesting happened.

Moments after being taken off the respirator, a miniscule movement was noted in Mr. Z.'s fingers. At first, we thought that we were hallucinating, but then it happened again.

We weren't sure initially what it meant. The neurologist felt that it might have been reflex movement. However, we decided to recommend that we place Mr. Z. back on the respirator and continue supportive care. The family concurred, but we told them that we didn't have much reason for optimism.

Smaller movements transformed into bigger ones in the next few days. Two weeks later, Mr. Z. was actually talking, and in three weeks, he was up in a chair! In one month, he was transferred to a rehab facility. We were awestruck and amazed.

I never have forgotten this case. It left an indelible impression on me. Here I was, a doctor, who was supposed to know the answers, giving the family no hope for their loved one's survival. I found out quickly how little I know, and it taught me that the ultimate power was not at all in my hands but emanated from a spiritual realm that I didn't understand.

Over the past twenty years, I have seen events such as this occur on several occasions, and I can only call them miracles. I'm sure that some might argue with me and offer scientific explanations for everything. I have learned, however, how little I know about life and death. I have definitely seen enough to know that no human being has the ultimate power to decide issues of life and death.

I am often asked how long a patient might have to live. I sometimes give the available statistics about a prognosis, but I always qualify my remarks by telling the patient and his or her family that only the Lord above has that answer. I have seen a lot of people beat the odds, and I know that I am not the dealer, nor is it my house.

A Candle in the Wind

I once knew a forty-two-year-old hardworking man with a wife and daughter. He was active and loved to work and play hard.

He usually worked twelve to fourteen hours a day and did this for years.

Charlie had asthma and used his inhalers frequently, but he never took the time to go to see a doctor. He was too busy doing things for other people, and he always put off taking care of himself.

One day, during an average day at work, an employee found Charlie sprawled on the floor of the bathroom in his office. I was at his side within a very short time and did cardiopulmonary resuscitation, or CPR, for two hours.

Nothing worked and eventually we "called the code" and pronounced him dead. Three doctors worked on him, and I could not bring myself to quit trying because I was his friend. The other two doctors convinced me that it was time. I just couldn't be objective enough to make this decision. Afterwards, I washed my hands in an attempt to rid myself of the stench of my friend's death, but I couldn't. No matter how hard I tried, it was in vain.

I had the terrible ordeal of breaking the tragic news to Charlie's wife and daughter, who were waiting for me in the family room. Tears welled in my eyes as I spoke, and I'm sure that the shock and horror of the ordeal could be read on my face.

I had nightmares about doing CPR on a man who was not only a fellow doctor and partner in my medical practice but also a close friend who had suddenly become my patient. I woke up with cold sweats for a long time after that fateful day. Charlie was more than just a friend. Like many of my other patients, he taught me as much in death as he had in life. He loved life and lived it to the fullest.

Charlie took care of everyone else, but he forgot to take good care of himself. He was a candle in the wind, one that burned at both ends. He left behind a family and much that was left undone. I refuse to walk down that path because I have too much to live for. It gave me another sad look at the ultimate finality of death and at my own mortality.

Endnotes

1. Blanchard, *The Heart of a Leader—Insights on the Art of Influence*, (Honor Books, 1999).

2. Covey, *The 7 Habits of Highly Effective Families*, (Golden Books, 1997).

3. Boisaubin, *Romancing the Patient: Boundary Issues in the Patient-Doctor Relationship*, UTMB, Galveston.

4. Vernon's Texas Statutes and Codes, Annotated Civil Statutes, Title 71, Chapter 6., Article 4495b, Medical Practice Act.

5. See Boisaubin.

6. Setness, "Patient Education by Proxy?" *Postgraduate Medicine*, Vol. 107, No. 6, May 15, 2000, p. 16.

7. Ibid.

CHAPTER 6

Death Be Proud

"You would know the secret of death.
But how shall you find it unless you
seek it in the heart of life?
The owl whose night-bound eyes are blind unto
the day cannot unveil the mystery of light.
If you would indeed behold the spirit of death,
Open your heart wide unto the body of life.
For life and death are one, even as the
river and the sea are one."

K. Gibran, *The Prophet*

Over the past twenty-three years, I have seen a lot of people pass from this life into the next. Some have been friends, some were loved ones, but most have been patients. Many have been both my friends and my patients. I have read about diseases and the stages of grieving over death. But what is written about death seems cold and impersonal next to the harsh reality of witnessing its effects in person.

There is no way to explain the helplessness and frustration that I have felt when I have seen families sob with grief as they learn of the death of a loved one. I will never forget the anguish that I have seen on the faces of people when I have told them that they have an incurable disease or that they are near death.

I have also seen incredible courage in the face of insurmountable odds; I have seen people with such strength of will that they are sapped of every ounce of strength and fortitude yet never give up until death literally steals their lives. The strength of human nature and its fortitude is never as indomitable as when it is tested under the direst of circumstances.

I have also seen people give up and feel that their death was a release from the bondage of their life. I have seen elderly people look me in the eye and tell me that they were at peace with themselves and ready to meet their maker. Some were certain that they were soon to see their loved ones in the hereafter and even welcomed death. Some were tired of fighting and needed to rest.

I have been trained to consider death as an enemy. However, I have discovered over the years that death is not always an evil force and that my job should not be to always fight it. There are times when I need to realize that all I can do is to ease the path along the final journey and that delaying it sometimes intensifies the pain of everyone involved.

Thoughts on "Physician-Assisted Suicide" and "Death with Dignity"

I am not going to debate the philosophical or religious aspects of death. I will leave that to the philosophers and theologians among us. However, I am qualified to discuss the impact of death on my patients and as it relates to me as both a human being and a doctor.

I have never taken death nonchalantly. Hell, most of us can't! I have been taught to fight it with everything in my professional arsenal, especially when it threatens to strike at children and young adults in the prime of their lives. I am forty-nine years old and have seen people die from diseases when they were "just too young to die." Cancer, heart disease, and accidents all cause such a tragic waste of life. I no longer think that I am invincible like I did when I was a teenage kid, when I didn't know any better and didn't have to look death in the eye.

There are times when I see so much suffering that I know deep down that my duty as a doctor is not to prolong life but to increase its quality. My experiences have convinced me that quality means more to most people than quantity. Most of my patients don't want to live to be one hundred years old unless, of course, they can be like George Burns and have a girl on each arm.

Physician-assisted suicide (PAS) violates and contradicts everything that a doctor stands for. It goes against the grain of spiritual and basic human principles that made me become a healer in the first place.

Anyone who has taken care of chronically ill patients knows that they experience periods of anger, depression, and isolation. They don't want to be a burden to others, and the decisions that they make are sometimes irrational or made under extreme duress. It is often difficult even for a trained doctor to know who is rationally capable of making this decision and who isn't. After all, we aren't talking about deciding where to vacation next year!

Psychological screening only helps so much. How do we know that a family member isn't pressuring mom or dad in order to reap the rewards of a last will and testament? Should we have enough faith in psychological testing to believe that it is infallible and that we should use it to allow patients to end their own lives?

As a doctor, I don't believe in artificially prolonging life when there is truly no hope for recovery. But, as you can see from the example of Mr. Z. in the preceding chapter, we don't always have the ability to know when that moment of irreversibility is. I am sure that God has reasons for not giving us the ability to know shades of gray when it comes to life and death.

Another consideration when we discuss PAS is that new methods of treatment and palliation are being found daily. How do we know that we won't cure an illness tomorrow or learn how to palliate its effects after we help someone die with it today? It is scary to think about where society is headed if PAS ever becomes accepted medical practice. PAS is reminiscent of Nazi Germany where people gave themselves absolute authority over life and death and physicians were given the ways and means to end life rather than to save it.

In the field of cardiology, I see people literally "come back from the dead," many of them to lead productive lives and to spend time with their families. No one can predict who can beat the odds, and that is why society should not expect or allow doctors to play God.

I have hated statistics since I was in college, probably because they seemed so cold and impersonal. They don't take into account the endurance of the human spirit or its strength of purpose. The medical literature is replete with statistics about the mortality rates of disease. I have made it my practice to no longer quote statistics about mortality, although many of my patients or their families pressure me to do so.

Doctors have to be able to handle this scenario. Scores of patients over the years have told me stories about how they had been "informed" by other doctors that they had only a few months or years to live. They beat the most terrible of odds. How can doctors be so wrong and so sure of themselves at the same time?

It is important to be both delicate and accurate when discussing a patient's prognosis with him or her or their family. People often "hear" what they chose to hear and often exaggerate the rest.

The line between life and death is often blurry. Our ability to define death is restricted to our limited understanding of what it really means, both spiritually and physically. We just don't understand the mystery that we call "death." As a doctor, I am not ashamed to admit that I have a limited grasp of the physical and spiritual concepts of death. More doctors need to admit their ignorance about this.

Some people say that a doctor's goal should be to allow people to die with dignity. But can we give dignity to something that is inherently without dignity?

> **"Death need not be dignified because it cannot be dignified. Death is an event, an occurrence that takes place in the normal course of human events. Death shows no partiality. It is not a 'thing' to be tamed because it has no being; it has no characteristics to be shaped or reformed.**
>
> **Much of the talk concerning 'death with dignity' is laden with false assumptions about what gives human beings value. Among these assumptions is that the manner of death one experiences is all that loved ones, family, and friends will remember about his or her death. Although a person's death can affect loved ones' memories of him, an entire life, with all of its contributions and meaning, cannot be dismissed and discounted even if the last days are spent tethered to a ventilator, tube-fed, diapered, or unable to recognize visitors."[1]**

Bedpans and IV poles surround most terminally ill patients. They are given intravenous or tube feedings and have tubes in their bladder, nose, and, sometimes, lungs. Private parts of the body are no longer sacred and are examined by nursing personnel, aides, and doctors.

Often patients can't control their bowels and other bodily functions. Usually they are connected to breathing machines or to a wide variety of support devices. There is nothing pretty about these sites, and many people prefer to die in familiar surroundings with their families present, without all the tubes and machines, and with the help of hospice care.

Hospice care has allowed doctors to follow the wishes of their patients while providing support and comfort for the entire family. It has given a sense of dignity to what otherwise is often a degrading experience. Terminally ill patients often choose to go home to die instead of staying in sterile (or sometimes dirty) hospital rooms where they are not in control of the situation. They want to be at home, in familiar surroundings, with their families nearby.

Hospice workers have provided incredible support for physicians, patients, and families at very difficult times by providing the important things that patients need so that they can die with some comfort, dignity, and control of their own fates. The truth is that doctors sometimes wait too long to recommend hospice care for their patients. The reason is probably that a lot of doctors are in denial when it comes to admitting that there is just nothing that they can do.

Numerous patients express the fear of being a burden to those around them. I have tried to help alleviate their anxiety and respect their "living will" instructions to be removed from life-prolonging equipment when the last vestige of hope is gone. I believe that it is their right to make that decision, and I honor their feelings because it is morally and ethically incumbent on me to do so.

Doctors routinely give pain medication and sedation to maintain the comfort of terminally ill patients. I don't think that anyone would argue that it is the humane thing to do. At times, when witnessing people who are in unbearable pain, it has been tempting to help them find an early end to their suffering. Being a doctor makes me even more sensitive to the suffering of others because it is my oath to do everything possible to prevent it. But what would happen if we gave doctors carte blanche to pull the plug or withdraw life support because these patients "weren't going to make it anyway?"

I agree with the premise that "protecting human life has been viewed as the central purpose of medicine."[2] I also feel that it is accurate to state that the…

> **"social sanctioning of physician-assisted suicide dismantles this tradition, giving physicians greater power over patients and undermining society's ability to protect them. The legalization of PAS irrevocably undermines basic premises of the doctor-patient relationship and the trust that is required for it to be maintained. It upsets a framework based on that trust and on a doctor not having so much power that he loses his ability to do what is truly in the patient's best interests.**
>
> **Can physicians kill patients upon request and return unaffected to the care of patients whose conditions are similar, but who chose not to die? How will the cancer patient who desires to live as long as possible view the physician who returns from a conference on the latest euthanasia techniques?"[3]**

We seem to have become confused over the terms "quality of life" and "dignity of death" when we should be using our empathy and humanity instead of meaningless terminology and statistics. What should a doctor's goals be when tending to the terminally ill? Should it be to give patients a quick end to pain and suffering, to prolong their lives with the latest technological advancements, or should our goal be to allow people to die with serenity and dignity surrounded by family and loved ones?

Will society become too concerned with money to want to keep dying people from using up valuable financial resources? We can't allow these answers to be determined by people who are followers of Hitler or Kevorkian. Both life and death can be respected at the same time that they are given both dignity and meaning. The sanctity of life cannot be sacrificed for the expediency or the economics of society.

Are Doctors Doing Enough to Assist the Terminally Ill?

The sad truth is that, while most doctors do not agree with PAS, many fail to provide adequate palliation of patients' symptoms before death. A disturbing article appeared in *The New England Journal of Medicine,* which states that suffering from pain is more likely in children suffering from cancer whose parents reported that the physician was not actively involved in providing end-of-life care.

Many physicians whose patients were in the study did not even report uncomfortable symptoms in their notes. The article goes on to state that:

"High-quality palliative care is now an expected standard at the end of life....Fatigue was the most frequently reported symptom and most of the children with fatigue suffered a great deal from it,

> according to their parents. Furthermore, there was little attempt on the part of clinicians to treat this problem. Our data suggest that there may be a lack of awareness among physicians that the suffering caused by certain symptoms typically experienced at the end of life may be amenable to palliation.
>
> For most children with cancer, the primary goal of treatment is to achieve a cure. Considerations of the toxicity of therapy, the quality of life, and growth and development are usually secondary to this goal. As a result, it may be difficult for physicians to change their focus even when there is little hope of a cure.
>
> We also found that earlier discussion of hospice care was associated with a greater likelihood that parents would describe their child as calm and peaceful during the last month of life.
>
> Of the children who were treated for specific symptoms, treatment was successful in 27 percent of those with pain and 16 percent of those with dyspnea (shortness of breath)."[4]

These findings are certainly disturbing. One has to wonder why doctors who are otherwise good clinicians would be lax in an area that is so critically important. A natural human response is to distance oneself from the dying patient. Some doctors are guilty of mentally "moving on" because they find more positive energy in taking care of a patient who has hope than in taking care of the dying. It takes strength to take care of those who are dying. It's easy to be around those who don't remind us of something unpleasant.

Watching people die is emotionally disturbing for everyone, but it is a sad fact of life. The compassion with which doctors deal with death and the dying is what matters to both patients and their families:

"To affect the quality of the day, that is the highest of arts."

Henry David Thoreau

Emotional Bonds—Right, Wrong, or Just Unavoidable?

One of the best professors of Oncology at Baylor College of Medicine taught me to avoid emotional connections with my patients. I was taught to keep a safe distance. His logic came from years of experience with the care of terminally ill patients.

He taught that it is important to not allow our patients to call us by our first names at any time. Maintaining objectivity is of paramount importance, and it's just not professional! He taught us that our objectivity is jeopardized by close personal relationships with patients. The relationship needs to be caring but impersonal.

One of my cancer patients once called me by my first name, and as an intern, this really didn't faze me. My professor overheard the remark and warned all of the interns and residents never to let their patients get emotionally close enough to them to be called by their first names: "Always correct a patient when he calls you 'Steve.'"

When I corrected my patient on the next go-around, his reaction shocked me. He looked betrayed and hurt. Our relationship changed suddenly, and he became withdrawn. I felt torn between what I had been taught and what I was feeling. What was right? My gut told me that being called by my first name was not all that bad a thing. Besides, I felt that I was being somewhat haughty and snobby by demanding to be called by my title.

Although I agree with my professor's basic premise, my own experience taught me that by correcting my patient's behavior, I changed the dynamics of our relationship. When he became withdrawn, it affected my ability to care for him. He needed to feel that I was his friend as well as his doctor. How could I take my friendship away from a man who was dying? It was something that comforted him during his last days, and when I admitted it to myself, it comforted me as well.

I later found that I could indeed protect my objectivity and my professionalism and still allow my patients to call me by my first name. I have certainly been called worse things as both a human being and as a doctor. The title itself is not as important as the relationships that I had created as a result of that title.

I have come to the understanding that emotional bonds are necessary and unavoidable both for myself and for my patients. It's hard to lovingly care for someone over a period of time without bonding emotionally with that individual. Sharing emotions such as joy and sadness with the people that surround us is as much an occupational hazard of the medical profession as is a needle stick. But doctors can use these emotions to become great doctors rather than just good doctors, or they can run away from them and become ineffective caregivers.

The "Backstroke," or the Avoidance Response to the Dying

Because of the personality that made me a doctor, I hate to admit defeat. I hate the concept that death has overcome my best efforts. Most doctors that I know share the dilemma of taking care of patients who defy our abilities. Our failure to alleviate suffering often stares us right in the face. Visits to patients' rooms often become shorter as the situation becomes more hopeless and more of the responsibility of care is passed onto others. Nurses and support personnel start to spend more time with the patient and family than the doctor as he moves onto others to whom he can offer more hope. It's also a way of avoiding and ignoring unpleasantness and the grim reminders of failure.

This dilemma often results in the doctor doing the "backstroke," which is a natural human response to something that most of us as human beings would rather avoid. It also puts the doctor out of touch with the patients who require his compassion, efforts, and skills more than ever. Doctors sometimes forget that suffering and dying patients require more time, strength, and energy than those who are more fortunate. What we find is sometimes a disappearing act, as the *NEJM* article unfortunately shows.

Doctors have it lucky in some respects. They don't have to stay at the patient's bedside and carry out countless orders, nor do they have to deal with an emotionally distraught family for more than a few minutes at a time. Nurses empty the bedpans and hospice workers take care of the nitty-gritty aspects of patient care. These people are left to offer compassion and support long after the doctor leaves the bedside.

A lot of doctors spend only a few minutes per patient on rounds. That is a pretty insignificant amount of time when you think about the daily problems of the terminally ill and dying. The "backstroke" is a dance step that most doctors do instinctively as a way of ignoring what they choose not to see.

Whether this reaction is due to the nature of a doctor's job, with all of its fatigue and pressures, or whether this relates to a reluctance to deal with emotionally charged and draining issues is a debatable point. Whatever the reason, the result is unfair to patients and their families.

My hat is off to those healthcare workers who stay at their patients' bedsides and deal with the unpleasantness of suffering without doing the "backstroke." They are the ones who touch the dying when they need to be touched. They embrace the tears and the sobs of families and friends with compassion and allow human beings to die with serenity and dignity.

My Early Experiences with Death

My first memories of death are vivid; the faces are as clear as if it all happened yesterday. I lost my first patient in the Cardiac Catheterization Laboratory quite unexpectedly.

Tom was a middle-aged male who had severe coronary heart disease. After a routine injection of his right coronary artery, he went into ventricular fibrillation. I shocked his heart over and over again and did CPR for an hour, but it seemed like an eternity. I could get no response from his heart. He succumbed despite all of our team's efforts.

I was angry and took this loss personally. For a time, I secluded myself in a room and just sobbed. Self-doubt entered my mind: "Am I as good a doctor as I thought?" I analyzed the case over and over again, asking myself if there was something that I should have done differently.

Blaming myself for his death, guilt caused me to question every move that I made. Depressed, I talked to the family and told them what had happened. They could probably tell how I felt by the look in my face; they consoled me almost as much as I consoled them.

It took me a long time to come to terms with this loss. How could this have happened to me? For the first time, I felt powerless over life and death, and it bothered me. I felt a sense of shame that death had gotten the upper hand. Tom's demise also made me recognize that what I did could both hurt as well as help people; I recognized the meaning of the saying: "Death defies the doctor or employs him to do its job."

I felt tortured over this case, but eventually my inner shame and self-doubts dissipated. This isn't the only patient that I have lost, but all of them had one thing in common: each of them was very sick and couldn't be saved from the fate that awaits us all. I had to develop a capacity to cope with death in order to survive. It was necessary for me to stop taking death "personally." Initially I developed a feeling of numbness that helped me cope with the sights and sounds of death. Later I recognized that there are certain basic truths about death that I had to learn for self-preservation:

- Death is inevitable for us all.
- No one can predict when it is someone's "time," although patients' premonitions often turn into reality, and doctors develop "a feeling" that death is imminent.
- No one, not even a doctor, can prevent it when the time has come, and
- Only God knows the answers to the mysteries that surround death.

Understanding these simple facts has given me comfort and has allowed me to be a better doctor and a healthier human being. But I needed more.

Coming to Spiritual Terms with Death

I have found it very difficult to deal with death on both a personal and a professional level. At times, I have even found myself doing the "backstroke" as a way of avoiding the pain associated with it. Death is a concept that has been difficult for me to grasp. But its specter keeps haunting me so that I can't shut it out for long, no matter how hard I try.

My defense mechanisms try to shut out the feelings of failure and inadequacy that I feel in death's presence. I have tried to understand death both physically and spiritually by reading about it, thinking about it, and praying over it. After doing all of these things, two things have become very apparent about death: I don't know much about it, and I have no power over it.

When I treat two people with the same illness with identical treatments, the outcomes are sometimes totally opposite. Does this happen because no two people are alike nor respond predictably because we are all unpredictable human beings? Or were my methods inadequate, and I was just lucky to have saved one of them? Is this evidence that there is a power greater than me that is in control of our destinies?

Out of necessity to maintain sanity, I have come to spiritual terms with death. That doesn't mean that I'm not afraid of it—quite the opposite; the thought of death terrifies me. It also forces me to make decisions that are based upon information that could be incomplete and is certainly not infallible.

I have discovered that it is difficult for me to deal with death, let alone comfort my patients, if I don't have inner peace and a strong sense of who I am. You can't buy either of these in a store or learn about them from a medical textbook. I have discovered a lot about inner peace in a book called the Bible, from my patients who are also my teachers, and from my family.

My inner peace comes from a strong belief in God and the knowledge that He walks with me in everything that I do. He is the doctor for my soul. God gives me strength to deal with death and the rest of life's difficulties and the courage and serenity to know what I can and cannot accomplish in life, both for myself and for my patients:

The Serenity Prayer

"God, grant me the serenity to accept the things that I cannot change, courage to change the things that I can, and wisdom to know the difference."

"The Serenity Prayer" has at times been my best friend, and it is often the best medicine that I can administer to my patients and to my own soul. It helps us enjoy our successes and deal with our failures, including the things that we cannot control: pain, suffering, and even death.

There is another very short verse that reminds me that my patients and I are never alone:

> **"Even tho I walk through the valley of the shadow of death, I will fear no evil; for thou art with me. Thy rod and thy staff, they comfort me."**

Psalm 23.4

I have read this verse since I was a child, but it has never meant as much to me as it has since I became a doctor!

Involving the Clergy as a Source of Strength and Support

People are most likely to realize the importance of their faith when they are down and out, when they have a severe debilitating illness, or when they face death. Many doctors shy away from dealing with spiritual issues with their patients. Some doctors are just uncomfortable with the subject of spirituality while some feel that it is an inappropriate topic for a medical conversation or an intrusion of privacy. Others just don't want to take the time for it!

It has been found in studies that religion not only decreases depression and suicide, but it also increases longevity.[5, 6] It is important that we ask patients how we can help them through the tough times in their lives.

This can be done without getting involved in religious preferences that can make a doctor feel uncomfortable. The questions and comments can be open-ended and unthreatening to all involved. The door needs to be left open to this important topic that is often ignored!

If a patient is one of the roughly 70 percent who feel that religion is important in their lives,[7] then we should consider involving the clergy in his or her care. Members of the clergy have been an invaluable ally in treating my ill patients and their families. They have provided as aspect of care that I have felt poorly equipped to handle.

When I was in medical school, I was never taught how to relate to the religious and spiritual side of my patients' problems. I was never exposed to clergymen, who have a lot that they can teach us as physicians and a lot that they can impart to our patients. It is a shame that only a small minority of doctors even bring up spiritual or religious issues with their patients. Most of us learned "to separate church and state" as part of our training.

Spiritual healing is an important part of treating the patient as a human being instead of as a set of biological cells. Doctors need to do better, but first they must address the question of why they are uncomfortable and insecure with these important issues. Are doctors afraid of treading on "personal" territory that makes them uncomfortable?

Doctors need to find a "comfort zone" with the concepts of religion and spirituality and understand their importance in the lives of their patients. They also need to incorporate these concepts into their own lives.

Premonitions

People often have a "sixth sense" and know when it is "their time." I have a bad feeling when a patient goes into a procedure with a premonition of her death. She is usually right.

God gives us feelings as warnings, and I have learned to take them seriously. When a patient has a heart attack and is about to "code," you can see it in her eyes and hear it in her voice. You know deep down that the patient's time is short. She knows it too.

It is scary when, prior to going into the Catheterization Lab, a patient tells me that she doesn't think she will survive the procedure. I have no doubt that our instincts are more than just mystical imaginings. We just sometimes ignore them because they aren't based on scientific reasoning. I have cancelled surgery based upon a patient's forebodings. I have seen enough to know that these premonitions are often surprisingly accurate and real.

Being a doctor has allowed me to develop heightened senses and an awareness of those around me. I can usually tell when my patients are near death's doorstep. A colleague, who is a nephrologist, sees so much death that he feels that he can predict the death of his patients to the day and even to the hour!

I won't pretend to play God or to know what His plans are for any of us, but I am certain that these feelings are given to us all for a reason. I think that God means for us to give these feelings special attention so that we can better care for each other.

It would be difficult for one to live the life of a doctor and truly feel that premonitions are mere coincidences.

Lessons from Death

The Valiant Fighter

I remember the words,
As I held back the tears.
They haunt me to this day.
Even after all these years,
Why do they affect me this way?

"There's much for which to live,
But you have so little time.
I wish I had more to you to give,
Tho' I vow to fight as if your life
Were mine."

My heart is heavy,
My mind is lost.
Your struggle with tragedy,
So valiant, but at great cost.

Such courage never before
Have I seen,
Your pain has shown me how
To live.

You surely are an evergreen,
To you everlasting life,
He will give.

No matter how much I hate to admit it, death has been my teacher. I have learned a lot about myself and about the people whom I have cared for due to death's presence. I have learned a lot about how to care for the living and about life itself because of death's teachings.

It has unfortunately taught me a lot about the unfairness and cruelty of life, as death stalks innocent victims without mercy. I have also seen death as a welcome friend to those who are withering on the vine with cancer and chronic illness: something not to be feared but an end to suffering. For some, it is a reunion with their loved ones.

I have seen examples of how to live life with courage, compassion, and strength, the likes of which I have never seen before. People who know they are going to die make every minute count. Why can't the rest of us? Do we need to know that the end is near to put our affairs in order and make things right with the people we love?

I have seen families brought closer together by death, and I have seen people develop an appreciation for things that cannot be counted in dollars and cents, such as the love of families and friends. The dying have no need of ambition and the merry-go-round of the material world that enslaves so many of us.

Death has most importantly taught me that we all need to have some form of spirituality to face both life and death. I know my limitations and that I am just an instrument of His will. I hope to be a messenger of comfort and peace rather than an instrument of death, but there is no way to know God's will in advance.

I often wish that I had a "retrospectoscope" to be able to undo my decisions if things went badly in surgery. Some patients could have lived shorter or longer lives if they didn't have the operation that I had suggested. My guilt has turned into an inner peace with the knowledge that death can be my teacher and that I can take lessons from the dying. It is said that:

"Once you learn how to die, you learn how to live."[8]

The most important thing that I have learned from death is that I am never alone, nor are my patients, as long as we have faith.

"For what is it to die but to stand naked in the
Wind and to melt into the sun?
For what is it to cease breathing but to free
The breath from its restless tides, that it may rise
And expand and seek God unencumbered?
Only when you drink from the river of silence
Shall you indeed sing.
And when you have reached the mountain top,
Then shall you begin to climb.
And when the earth shall claim your limbs, then
Shall you truly dance."

K. Gibran, *The Prophet*

A Doctor's Reflections on the Preciousness and Sanctity of Life

I have seen people die who are younger than me. Several of my friends have committed suicide during my years of training. A partner who practiced closely with me died suddenly while seeing patients in our office.

All of these events occurred without warning. What these people had in common was the fact that death took them in the prime of their lives and left their families without their loved ones way too early.

As a doctor, I have studied the physiology of death. Cells start to die, brainwaves disappear, and the heart stops beating. I have asked God over and over again to explain the deeper meaning of death to me so that I could have a better understanding of why people die when they seemingly shouldn't.

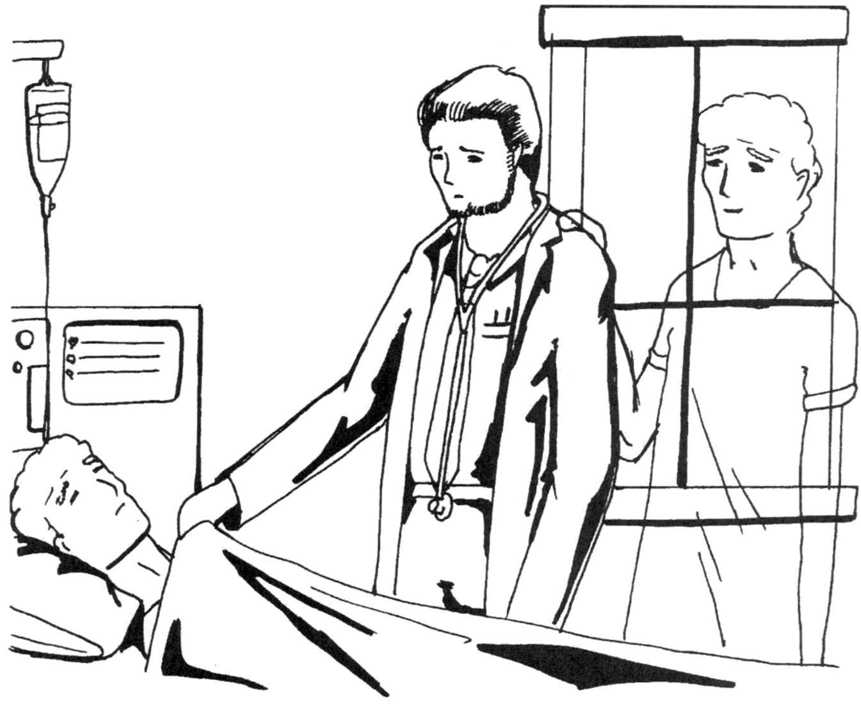

Being a doctor allows me to experience more of death firsthand than, fortunately, most people see. But I have also seen its cold reality as a human being; it has taken the lives of those who are close to me and younger than me. I hate not knowing why, and it tests the limits of my faith in God to try to understand something that I know I will never understand.

A lesson from death is that life is precious. We can't take it for granted. Every moment should be treasured because tomorrow is not promised to any of us. I have seen the unfair face of death as a doctor and know that it could strike any of us at any time.

Heart disease is my specialty. It is one of the cruelest of death's weapons. It comes in stealth, hidden in shadows, and often claims its next victim without regard to age or fairness. My mission to defeat death often ends in tears of sadness, but sometimes it ends in tears of happiness and thankfulness to God for granting a loved one at least one more day to be with his or her family.

If I cheat death, I know that it is only temporary victory. It will continue to stalk its prey. I know deep down that God has plans for all of us and that when it is our time, there is nothing that anyone can do to alter the inevitable. But until then....

Being a doctor has taught me how fragile and sacred life really is. Death has taught me a lot about how to live.

Endnotes

1. Blocher, *The Right to Die? Caring Alternatives to Euthanasia* (Chicago, Moody Press, 1999), p. 57.

2. Ibid.

3. Ibid.

4. Wolfe et al, "Symptoms and Suffering at the End of Life in Children with Cancer," *New England Journal of Medicine*, Vol. 342, No. 50, p. 326.

5. Larson and Koenig, "Is God Good for Your Health? The Role of Spirituality in Medical Care," *The Cleveland Clinic Journal of Medicine*, Vol. 67, No. 2, Feb. 2000, p. 80.

6. Ibid.

7. Ibid.

8. Albom, *Tuesdays with Morrie, An Old Man, a Young Man, and Life's Greatest Lesson* (Doubleday, 1997), p. 82.

CHAPTER 7

Of Butterflies and Men

"Caterpillar
Brown and furry
Caterpillar in a hurry,
Take your walk
To the shady leaf, or stalk,
Or what not,
Which may be the chosen spot.
No toad spy you,
Hovering bird of prey pass by you;
Spin and die,
To live again a butterfly."

Christina Rossetti

Changes and Awakenings

Some of the most beautiful things in life are a result of "change": A caterpillar changes into a gorgeous butterfly, the inspiration of Rossetti's poem. Ice melts into water that, in turn, fills picturesque lakes and rivers. We read fairy tales about frogs changing into handsome princes. Transformation is more than just a figment of our imagination. Our lives are full of change; we read about it, but for some reason, we are afraid of it, and we often try our best to avoid it.

The fear of "change" could be described in the following way:

> **"We cling tenaciously to our habitual ways of doing things, thinking they are our only choices. We may resist anything new or different through indecisiveness. We waver, going back and forth between fear and doubt, fear that change will be painful, doubt that it will make a difference in our lives."[1]**

Our bodies change on a day-to-day basis. We either ignore it or try our best to fight it; none of us wants to grow old. We don't have a choice when it comes to aging, at least not yet. In a sense, we are all caterpillars waiting to come out of our cocoons, but it is difficult for most of us to see the natural beauty that accompanies the aging process. It is fashionable to fight nature; society teaches us to try to stay young. We even go to the doctor to look younger through plastic surgery. We don't want to come out of our protective cocoons and accept change in our lives.

In my case, it took the pain and despair of my life to see that I needed a more powerful physician, one who could heal my spirit and my body and help me to do the things that were necessary and important for my health and happiness. As you can tell from prior chapters, I had done an awful job of trying to be my own doctor. It was not a healthy experience, and it led to a cycle of perpetual failure, depression, and unhappiness.

A princess may not have kissed me, but I was touched by a King. And it was not a fairy tale. I would like to tell you the story of my own spiritual journey and how being a doctor has helped awaken me to the true wonders of life.

Wandering in the Desert for Forty Years (Without Moses)

When I think back on the first four decades of my life, I realize that I accomplished a great deal but that I was also unhappy and confused with my goal-oriented focus on life. I was hell-bent on becoming a great doctor (not just a good doctor), and I lost sight of everything else that was important in the process.

I thought that I had all the answers and that I didn't need help from anything or anybody. After all, I was my own man! Medicine was my highest priority, as well as the most time consuming, and everything else took a back seat.

I had nurturing parents and a strong sibling rivalry with my sister who later became a successful attorney and judge. My parents placed a high priority on success, as you have read in earlier chapters. They taught me right from wrong and have given me strong moral values. I didn't always listen, and I rebelled against them and most everything that they stood for. It has only been in recent years that I have come to an understanding of the source of this rebellion.

I rebelled inwardly, if not outwardly, against organized religion. I went to Hebrew School for five years, not only on

Sundays but also after public school three afternoons a week. I did all the things that custom and tradition demanded from a Jewish boy, and I had my Bar Mitzvah at the traditional age of thirteen when Jewish boys suddenly become "men" and accept the responsibilities of adult leadership.

Inwardly, I followed these rituals in order to appease my parents and to make them happy. Anything less than graduating into manhood by my thirteenth birthday would have been a disappointment to my family and friends and would have alienated me from the Jewish community that gave me my identity.

I felt no special relationship with God during these years, and I mechanically went through the motions to follow my religion's traditions, many of which I now recognize as being beautiful. But at that stage of my life, they represented an albatross that my parents and ancestors placed around my neck. It was something that I didn't particularly want or need. It was a burden that I felt was unfair, but I accepted it, at least superficially.

As I grew older and reached my twenties, my rebellion became more blatant. I made my parents cringe by dating non-Jewish women, and I flaunted a lifestyle that was alienated from religion in general, and that often alienated me from my family.

God became superfluous. I didn't need religion in my life; everything that I needed to know could be explained in a test tube or in a science lab. Anything else was unimportant or unnecessary. My goals were clear, and I left Judaism by the wayside.

As an English major, I read a lot during my college years. I read Nietzsche and Sartre along with many great writers and philosophers. Existentialism and religion just didn't mix, and it was much more socially acceptable to read the former, and much better for my grades. So I chose Nietzsche. I also chose Shakespeare and Freud because they opened up a whole new world for me. I felt enlightened in the "think tank" of college.

My required reading list didn't include *The Bible*. I chose to look in other directions and refused to go to more Hebrew School after my Bar Mitzvah. Religion was a memory, and I didn't want it to be part of the present or future.

I wanted to be like Nietzsche and make my own bold choices and shape my life. I had lived the guilt of *Portnoy's Complaint* for most of my young life, and I desperately wanted to expand my horizons and escape my guilt at the same time. To me, religion epitomized guilt and pressure rather than peace and security.

Like a lot of young people who know what is best for them, I ignored my parents' advice; as a matter of fact, I usually went the opposite direction. In retrospect, I rebelled in an attempt not only to escape the suffocating strictness of religion but also to establish a name for myself, the younger brother.

Having a successful older sister generated a lot of insecurities. I was supposed to follow in her successful footsteps but chose instead to do something very different for myself. I needed to break the cast-iron mold into which I felt I had been poured. Instead, I almost escaped into oblivion.

I went through college and med school thinking that religion was hypocritical. I attended services during the high holidays of Rosh Hashanah and Yom Kippur and sometimes during Passover and Hanukah. I secretly enjoyed Passover Seders and reading *The Four Questions* although I didn't want to admit it to myself or to anyone else, for that matter.

I have fond memories of searching for Hanukah "gelt" and of lighting candles although it wasn't as much fun as I imagined that my Christian friends were having lighting their Christmas trees. I always felt that they had the better end of the deal! I couldn't break away from Judaism altogether. There was too much of Portnoy's guilt in me for that and too much of a feeling of obligation to my family and people.

You have read about the emotional, marital, and financial carnage that followed me after I finished school. If I had set out to prove something to myself, the results weren't anticipated.

What I wound up proving was that I had rejected something that was very important to my life, all because I was too stubborn to admit that I couldn't do it all by myself. I needed help, but pride got in the way!

There had been a void in my life since I was very young. I never realized it until I was a lot older, rid myself of the camouflage, and forced myself to take a hard look in the mirror. It took quite a long time for me to understand where my feelings of emptiness came from. I couldn't find the answers by myself. In order to find my way out of the abyss that had become my life, I had to realize that there was something missing and that my answers couldn't be found by hiding from myself.

I was alone and wandering, and no matter how hard I tried, I couldn't find a compass that would point me in the right direction. Although I was outwardly successful, I was inwardly a lost soul. My life gradually became a puzzle that couldn't be solved. All the pieces were there in front of me, but I didn't know how they fit together.

I maintained the façade of the successful physician, but beneath the surface, I barely held things together. My inner turmoil was reflected by the repeated failures of my personal life. I knew that I was a successful doctor on the surface, but I really had no idea **who** I was.

I was searching for a way to fill the emptiness that I felt wrenching at the pit of my stomach, something that threatened to tear apart my soul. I felt incomplete and didn't know where to go or which way to turn. I didn't want to admit that I needed a Higher Power to show me the way.

Looking for the Promised Land

If you remember your Bible stories, the Jews were a proud and obstinate people who at times worshiped false idols instead of the one true God. They strayed from God's commandments, in spite of everything that He did for them, and were denied "the promised land" until they were deemed worthy. Before *The Chosen* were given their home, they were a rebellious and sometimes arrogant lot.

My life ran in parallel to this biblical chapter of *Exodus*. God taught me about Moses and His commandments when I was very young, but I chose to worship false idols instead. I was rebellious, headstrong, and sometimes arrogant, just like my forefathers. I worshipped the material successes of life and cared little about God or His teachings.

There was no sudden event that made me realize what God was doing with my life, no sudden hammer blow that knocked sense into me. It took years and a series of important events and people to make me understand that God was trying to prepare me for something that I didn't comprehend. He did this by hitting me over the head repeatedly until I begged for mercy.

It wasn't until later that I realized that God had filled my life with blessings that I didn't appreciate. I had three beautiful children, generally in good physical health; and I was blessed with a fulfilling career that helped other people. All of this was lost in my unhappiness and feelings of emptiness and isolation.

God put certain people, places, and events in my life that nudged me, sometimes not so gently, along the way. You are aware of some of the self-induced tragedies in my life; now its time to hear the other side of the story.

The Celestine Prophecy

James Redfield's famous novel talks about "coincidences" as:

"happening more and more frequently and that, when they do, they strike us as beyond what would be expected by pure chance. They feel destined, as though our lives had been guided by some unexplained force."[2]

This is the first "insight," and it was also an insight for me personally.

A friend of mine gave me Redfield's book as a birthday present; I'm sure it wasn't a coincidence! Reading *The Celestine Prophecy* made me stop and think. I am far from being a mystic because of my science-oriented background. But there was a lot happening around me that I couldn't easily explain.

Deep down, I felt that other forces were at work. Over time, I became wise enough to know that I didn't understand very much about life. My youthful pride eventually evolved into a gradual understanding of the events that shaped my life.

I came to the realization that a lot of so-called random events were not at all coincidental. There were purposes and meanings behind them. I had to allow myself to be open-minded and to look at things on more than a superficial level.

New ideas and new people had to be allowed into my life. I couldn't learn any of this from a medical textbook or in a classroom; I had to observe things around me, sometimes seeing things as if for the first time.

All people have blind spots. For example, we often don't notice that the people who cross our paths may be there for a reason. Does life consist of absolute randomness?

If you have read the preceding chapters closely, you will understand that being a doctor has changed my life by placing certain people in my path at certain times. Certain events have transpired in order to reshape my thinking and increase my understanding of my place in the world around me.

Many "coincidences" have occurred while writing this novel. I have come across books and people who have given me food for thought at exactly the right moments. I have opened my eyes and my heart to their inspirations.

We are blind unless we allow ourselves to see and learn from others. It's our choice!

A Cardiologist and a Broken Heart

I have considered myself a good physician, but sometimes my ego would carry this a step further. Time has allowed me to see my strengths and weaknesses, and it has given me a better perspective of my role as a physician.

My experiences in life have taught me that there is but one true Healer who has ultimate power over life and death, happiness and suffering. I am a messenger who is sent to do His will and to pass on a gift that was given me to help others.

I had to first rid myself of any belief that I had the ultimate control over people's fates and destinies, even though my pride made that difficult and science had led me to believe that I could understand most things in the universe.

Treating thousands of patients has taught me that although my role is very important, it's not as important in the scheme of things as I originally thought. I have realized how little I actually know as I've grown older!

There are mental and physical illnesses that I just can't cure and that cannot be cured by any human physician. People have jokingly asked me if I could cure a broken heart. As a cardiologist, I realize that I am powerless against the most common heart disease known to man, and the most painful!

I have learned to treat my patients with every possible weapon at my command and then to hand things over to God. This gave me relief from my self-inflicted torment that came from failure.

I have also learned to "let go" of my own personal problems and to put them in God's hands. I can't be my own doctor; you've seen that this doesn't work. I have learned to put my problems, and those of my patients, in the hands of a higher power. That is the only way that I could become a truly good physician.

My Greatest Teachers

"The teacher who walks in the
shadow of the temple,
Along with his followers, gives not
of his wisdom but
Rather of his faith and lovingness."

K. Gibran, *The Prophet*

I have gone to school and trained for a total of twenty-five years. Countless teachers have crossed my path, some good and some bad, some memorable and some forgettable. I didn't always appreciate the good ones until much later. That was especially the case with my parents, whose values I didn't appreciate during my youth.

Like a lot of young people, I thought that my parents represented the old way of doing things. I didn't appreciate the love and nurturing affection that they gave me until much later, nor did I understand that they were responsible for the loving and caring nature that has made me a good doctor. They also taught me what it means to sacrifice for others by the way that they sacrificed for me.

I had to make my mistakes in life to realize that a lot of what they said had merit. What I am in life as a person is largely due to them.

My medical professors taught me the importance of knowledge but not much about life. My patients have been my greatest teachers, giving me lessons constantly about life and about death. They have also taught me about humility and about the fact that people often need to be weak before they can become strong.

My family has taught me a lot about love. They have taught me about being given second, third, or fourth chances and that failure isn't necessarily permanent, unless you allow it to be.

Medicine doesn't allow you to always be there for the important events in your children's lives. I would be proud if the initials "M.D." after my name stood for "My Daddy" because I would rather my children think of me as "Dad" than as "my father, the doctor." My children have taught me a lot about unconditional love, and I want to leave them a legacy of love in return.

God's love is like that of a parent for his child. It is as unswerving as is His forgiveness. The true power of grace entered my life because of my weaknesses. I know now that God was bringing me closer to Him through my failures and hardships.

It took forty years of wandering in the desert to be ready to accept His teachings for my family, my patients, and myself. I feel like the prodigal son who returned home to find love and to be healed (Luke 15: 11–32).

Lost and Found

One of my favorite Bible stories is *The Parable of the Prodigal Son*. I was lost and then found through the love of God and His son, Jesus. I have been baptized as a Christian although much of my blood is filled with a Jewish heritage that I love.

I consider the Jewish people to be my own, and they are always in my heart. Their blood is filled with the beauty of an ancient heritage, and they are God's "Chosen People." I feel a strong bond with them because I grew up with their teachings and traditions; they are my identity.

God revealed my own path by bringing special people into my life and allowing me to see the miracles that have been revealed to me as a doctor. He gave me the opportunity to finally study the greatest and oldest book of all.

God did bring me to my knees, but then he made me stronger through faith and love. The emptiness that I had felt in my life was replaced by His love. His grace and forgiveness have allowed me to forgive myself and to love myself.

I came to realize not only that I couldn't do it alone but that I was not alone. God is with me every hour of every day, not just when I wear my white coat. I no longer feel isolated and all alone in a world that at times is beautiful and at other times, sad, ugly, and cruel.

My spirituality and my faith have been my salvation from the pain that surrounds my life. I have also learned the importance of appreciating the beauty that surrounds me that I had never truly seen before.

God's love is a much more powerful medicine than anything that man can offer. It provides an inner peace and tranquility that I needed both to be healed and to allow me to effectively heal others. But I had been blind to it for so long!

I have a sense of who I am because of God's love. I feel a peace in my soul that is like the peace that I see in nature, a peace that I had found so elusive because I was looking for love in "all the wrong places."

But I know that I am human. I am going to make a lot more mistakes in my life, and I am far from perfect as a man or as a doctor. All I can do is pray and hope that God shows me the paths in life that He desires me to follow. Nancy Snyderman describes healing as a process in her recent book, *Necessary Journeys*:

"The first step toward healing is the admission that you can't, for the moment, go it alone. The second step is understanding that admitting you can't go it alone and getting help for yourself aren't signs of weakness but of resilience. Thinking yourself worthy of saving, of help, of change, is the beginning of the path. The final step is understanding fully and honestly that becoming whole is a process, not a lesson learned in hours or days; I still consider myself a work in progress."[3]

For some, healing involves counseling. For me, it took God's grace and love in addition to the help of very special friends that He put in my life. The truth is that no matter how many people offer their counseling and support, it takes a much stronger relationship to make the others work: a relationship with God.

I can now stop and laugh at myself and put my life in some perspective. An unbearable burden has been lifted off my shoulders because I know that I am not alone. I can also accept and like myself as less than perfect, in spite of my faults. I am no longer afraid of the reflection in the mirror or hide behind the white coat. I look in the mirror and see someone who is loved by the Father of all. After all, if God loves me, why shouldn't I love myself?

I certainly am far from being "off the hook" when it comes to blame and accountability. I feel even more accountable to those around me and to God than I felt before, but the difference is that now I don't take my failures and weaknesses as a human being personally.

When things don't go well with my patients or with my personal life, I ask myself if I did the best that I could and if I did the "right thing." If I can truthfully say "yes," then I can live with myself because I realize that the events of my life are determined by a higher power. I am here to help others if they can be helped. But I have learned that the decisions made from above are final, and I don't argue with the umpire like I did before.

I have lived through four divorces, a bankruptcy, financial disasters, embezzlement, and personal illness. I don't feel sorry for myself. Quite to the contrary, I consider myself a very lucky man. Being a doctor has taught me that my personal hardships are miniscule compared to the suffering of others. I consider myself blessed by a special ability that He has given me to help others, and I want to make the most of it while I'm here on earth.

I feel a special closeness with my parents who never stopped loving and supporting me. My father died two years ago, but I know that he is up in heaven looking down on me, and I know that I have a guardian angel up above who is taking care of me.

God has opened my eyes to the realization that there are many ways of helping others. There is a universe full of opportunities if we don't waste them.

I know now that there is an answer to the hell that I see every day around me, which had previously made me feel so helpless and depressed. I know that my dying patients are about to experience a beauty that I can't even imagine.

I have seen incontrovertible evidence in my daily life that God is both with me and with my patients. I have seen too much not to realize that I both appreciate and need Him. Today's miracles are often overlooked and unrecognized; they are not just chance happenings or "coincidences." Anyone who needs proof that miracles still happen every day of our lives should spend a day walking in the footsteps of a doctor.

There are several morals to this story. First, we shouldn't be afraid of change because it is part of the natural order of things. Transformation is the way that we grow and mature as individuals; we can't avoid it, deny it, or stop it.

What we often fail to realize is that change can help us unleash our inner beauty and help us appreciate the beauty that surrounds us. Change ought not be feared, but we struggle against it because we feel comfortable in our individual niches in life, and it is hard, even if we are unhappy, to try something new. This takes courage.

Secondly, faith in a supreme being is essential for us to accomplish change and to find inner peace. It doesn't matter if that faith is in a Christian, Jewish, Moslem, Hindu, or Buddhist God. A doctor needs to have faith in a higher power if he is to heal both himself and others.

Change

When we change, do we
Merely rearrange
The furniture? Or do we just move
Things around to feel more secure?

Changing, rearranging,
We spend so much of our lives
Clinging to the past,
Staying tied to it steadfast.

True change takes courage and bravery,
Not camouflage and trickery.
Self-deception is not the way,
Changing our lives requires us to pray.

Believing in the Lord is the
Strength that we need.
Being with him is to succeed in both death
And in life,
And gives peace without eternal strife.

Despite the numerous hardships that it put in my path, or maybe because of them, medicine enabled me to find both my God and myself. I was shown the miracles of life and death through both my own pain and suffering and by being a witness to the suffering of others.

Being a doctor made a believer out of me. But God turned me into a healer.

Endnotes

1. Brussat and Brussat, *Spiritual Rx, Prescriptions for Living a Meaningful Life*, (Hyperion, 2000), p. 247.

2. Redfield, *The Celestine Prophecy* (Warner Books, 1993).

3. Snyderman, *Necessary Journeys—Letting Ourselves Learn from Life*, (Hyperion, 2000), p. 122.

CHAPTER 8

Strategies for Healing

Many people have written about various aspects of what I am about to discuss. However, I would like to talk about several strategies that, in my experience, have proven themselves to be invaluable to the welfare of my patients. I have a slightly different perspective compared to others because of my own experiences as a patient with doctors and treatment programs.

I am going to discuss these strategies with the premise that healing involves making a person feel whole, both physically and spiritually. Healing doesn't involve a single avenue or approach. It is a two-way street between doctor and patient and hopefully leads us to realistic goals that we set for ourselves. Some of the roads are not paved or well traveled. Sometimes we have to be pioneers and experiment to see what works. There is no cookbook to follow; some things just make sense, and we have to follow our instincts and "gut feelings."

"An Ounce of Prevention"

My mother taught me my first lesson about medicine early on as a youngster. The old motto, "an ounce of prevention is worth a pound of cure," was said with an exclamation point in her voice every time she saw me play out in the snow of New Jersey's winters without wearing my hat and gloves.

We take our cars for oil changes to prevent engine problems, but most of the time, we treat our bodies with neglect and disrespect. We check the condition of our heaters and air conditioners more often than we go to the doctor's office for a physical exam.

Prevention has not been emphasized adequately in training programs for doctors although it has become much more popular and important in the public's eyes. We are taught how to diagnose and treat disease as physicians, but our education shortchanges us when it comes to learning how to keep people healthy and prevent disease in the first place.

There were few courses that taught methods of prevention in my training, and often the subject was totally ignored by professors. We learned that cholesterol was bad and that there were medications to keep it low, but we were never taught about other approaches to maintaining a healthy lifestyle. Admittedly, some of these ideas have become popular only recently as public awareness has increased.

We have a much more educated public that has forced doctors to learn how to take preemptive attacks against disease. Patients demand, and rightfully so, that we take the lead in preventing cancer, heart disease, and a variety of other illnesses. Public health has also made us much more aware of the importance of prevention with the AIDS epidemic.

We are living in the age of the Internet, which gives us the tools of a public library right in our very own homes. Public awareness now gives doctors no choice but to keep up with current trends and improvements in technology. We cannot afford to stay in the Stone Age while our patients educate themselves in areas of medicine and leave us behind in the dust.

People generally want to be healthy and to live longer, and now they have the technology to not only keep up with a lot of what their doctors are learning but also sometimes to get a step ahead of them. It's an embarrassing admission, but I have had to work hard to stay in a position of being an authority to my patients in preventive cardiology by keeping up with not only my reading material but theirs as well.

Patients often amaze me with questions and comments that reflect their ability to educate themselves about their problems. However, they still look to me as their doctor to be the ultimate authority on how to treat and prevent their diseases; they look for direction. If I don't know the answers as their doctor, I had better find another place to hang my shingle.

Preventive medicine is cost effective and necessary in today's environment of cost containment. For doctors, there may be a reluctance to spend a lot of time on prevention because insurance companies don't emphasize it in their reimbursement schedules. We need to change the priorities of the insurance industry and our own as doctors. We need to provide what society needs and demands. We need prevention rather than intervention. It's just good medicine to fight disease and to fight the spiraling costs of health care.

The Importance of Being Proactive

I like it when my patients are proactive and self-motivated. Contrary to my fears, this trait makes my job easier rather than more difficult.

As patients work on their own behalf, they sometimes become more demanding, but that helps keep me on my toes. It makes me work even harder when patients expect more out of me.

I am also a patient, which allows me to see both sides of the coin. Over the years, I have learned that perseverance is essential in finding the answers to my own problems. Usually nobody will hand these answers to me on a silver platter.

Some doctors feel insecure when their patients take an active role in their own care. They need to come to terms with their own insecurities and know that the old world where patients were passive is long gone. There is no question that we are far better off now than we were even ten years ago. We need to allow our patients to be a quarterback in the huddle and not just force them to sit on the bench while we call all the plays.

Patients need to demand to be in the huddle. If the doctor balks, then they need to simply find another coach, one who is open-minded and proactive and willing to look at a variety of alternatives, even if they are outside the traditional realm of medical care.

Motivational Techniques

Sometimes I wish that I had taken a course in motivational speaking. It would be great for a doctor to learn how to change apathetic, unmotivated patients into proactive people who are willing to work on their own behalves. It isn't always easy to find ways to motivate people; we are all very different. That is why I appreciate it when my patients come through the door ready to tackle and solve their problems, allowing nothing to get in their way.

I have learned several ways to motivate people to help themselves. One of the keys to motivation is trying to understand what makes people tick. Everyone is different in that regard. What motivates some will not motivate others.

I came to the realization long ago that spouses carry a lot more power than I ever could hope for. Enlisting spousal support in my efforts is crucial for a lot of my patients. Wives especially have ways of "convincing" their husbands to follow medical advice. The power of female persuasion should never be underestimated! After all, it's been with us since Adam and Eve. And it's important to have the wife on your side!

It is great for spouses to do things with their mates, such as exercising and dieting. It is hard for one partner to quit smoking or to follow a dietary or exercise program while the other is eating all that he or she wants and continuing to fill the room with cigarette smoke. I usually encourage spouses to enter programs together. It is healthy and motivational for them both.

It is important to set reasonable and realistic goals! No patient is going to get excited about following a strict diet or exercise regimen that doesn't provide tangible rewards. I encourage a rewards system. Usually this consists of allowing my patients a good, hearty steak dinner every so often, allowing them to eat their favorite unhealthy food as a reward for following the game plan. Doing anything without a break is boring and leads to eventual noncompliance in all of us. It's just human nature.

I also encourage financial and personal incentives. People need to understand that healthy living is cheaper in the long run than continuing to smoke, take medications, and live an unhealthy life. I would encourage the government to offer some economic incentives, such as tax breaks, to people who go to their doctor regularly and who practice good prevention in their homes.

It is important for my patients to witness my own tenacity and perseverance in their care. The idea is to get them motivated by seeing that I am motivated on their behalf. I try to set the example for them to follow. I tell them about the positive results of hard work and perseverance, but they have to see it for themselves.

- That extra half mile of effort pays off in the long run. I can't count how many times persistence has enabled me to open closed arteries that were remaining stubbornly closed. If I had given up easily, the end result would have been less than an optimal result for the patient. It pays to try hard and see just how "good it gets." I wouldn't want to go to a doctor who was a quitter.

I have also realized that you can "lead a horse to water, but you can't make him drink." Some people can't be motivated, and there may be other forces at work.

At times there are spiritual issues and psychological issues, including depression, that need to be dealt with before any other problems can be solved.

Spirituality and Prayer

Over the last twenty years, I have learned to value the spiritual side of healing. I refrain from forcing my beliefs on anyone, but I recognize that most people have some beliefs and that these beliefs are important in their healing process. The term "spirituality" means different things to different people. As a doctor, I feel it is important to keep an open mind. Perhaps my Jewish background has sensitized me to persecution and to the importance of respecting the beliefs of others.

It has been shown in a variety of studies that people who attend religious services regularly and have strong faith in God suffer less from depression, addiction, and high blood pressure and actually live longer than those who don't have a strong spiritual base in their lives.[1] The data definitely supports the role of faith in a supreme being as a strong promoter of physical and mental health.

I respect and encourage the need for patients and their families to pray, no matter what their beliefs. When appropriate, I actually ask them to pray for me as their doctor as well as with me for their loved ones. On many occasions, I have asked a religious leader to facilitate communication with the family. There is no doubt in my mind that having strong beliefs in a supreme being is important for patients' recovery. They also appreciate a doctor who respects these beliefs.

It is essential to remember that healing is helping someone to feel "whole." Doctors can heal their patients even without curing them. Doctors need to become increasingly aware of patients' cultural, social, and spiritual needs to feel well and respect them as an integral part of their medical care.

From my own experience, it is very difficult to see how doctors can heal their patients if they are not healthy themselves. It is difficult to fill another person's tank if ours is running on empty. It is important for our society to produce healthy doctors and not just concentrate on the patients that they treat. Training programs have often neglected this vital need, often sending book-smart but otherwise unhealthy and mentally unprepared doctors out into the real world.

Utilizing the Mind-Body Connection

Sometimes, as doctors, we tend to forget that people have heads attached to their bodies. We often look at a human being as a "textbook case" of this or that or as riddles that need to be solved. Life is a lot more complicated than that, and so are patients.

We are just learning about the interactions between body and mind. Courses are now being offered to doctors in this subject, and books are being written about how healing is affected by such things as meditation, humor, psychological state of mind, and spirituality. As doctors, we need to become sensitive and knowledgeable about these interactions because they are important to our patients.

Patients comment that they appreciate humor in a doctor. After all, doctors have a reputation for being kind of dull and boring people who only know how to talk about a single subject. Right, you guessed it! I actually go out of my way to socialize with people who are not doctors because I need to escape from my world into theirs. A lot of doctors live and breathe medicine. After a while, I can't listen to medical talk anymore!

To escape mental fatigue, I try to find humor in seemingly silly things. I like to encourage my patients to laugh at things that are sometimes outrageous or absurd; sometimes they are things that some people may not find funny. It helps both of us get a fresh outlook on things.

For example, I once took care of a morbidly obese female who weighed 750 pounds. She came to my office with her stomach calloused from being dragged on the floor in front of her when she walked. When she sat, no one could see her legs or feet. Part of my physical exam called for me to exam her lower extremities for edema. Since I could not see them due to the pounds of flesh in front of her hiding them from view, I crawled under her chair for this part of the examination. I did this in a rather dramatic fashion, crawling on all fours around and under her chair. She recognized my difficulty, and we both started laughing.

This was an unusual and hilarious situation, and she was able to laugh at herself and at her own physical problems. We were able to laugh together at something that would have looked absurd to anyone around us. The alternative was for her to feel isolated and depressed, which certainly would not have helped her.

You can't expect people to always be able to laugh at their infirmities and at themselves. Cancer and heart disease are anything but funny, but sometimes you just have to find small things to laugh at in order to be able to deal with the big picture. More importantly, I have had to learn how to laugh at life and at myself in order to maintain my own sanity. I have tried to help my patients see the humor in the seemingly ridiculous situations that we share.

My patients often rely on me to set the mood, but there are times when they have lifted me out of depression by their humor and upbeat mood. It really does work both ways. They affect me as much as I affect them, "for better or for worse."

I would like to discuss two other examples of the mind-body connection. Smoking cessation and stress are examples of important mind-body interactions that are encountered in the daily practice of medicine. They represent two of the biggest challenges to the welfare of my patients, and they are two of the most frustrating problems that I have had to deal with as a doctor.

I have the power and knowledge to combat disease, to open arteries with balloons and stents, but I am utterly powerless when it comes to convincing many of my patients to quit smoking. Lectures are often meaningless about the terrible risks of smoking and its association with lung cancer and heart disease. People have heard it all before in the news media, but somehow they just can't bring themselves to quit.

Because of nicotine's strong addiction potential, many people can't break the habit, even with the help of modern smoking-cessation medications, acupuncture, or hypnosis. It certainly comes down to "mind over matter." A lot of my patients realize that they are killing themselves, but they still can't quit. It is frustrating to watch a person self-destruct. I feel like the mechanic who works on the car, oiling the gears and fine-tuning the engine, only to have the driver go out of the garage and be careless.

Stress is another killer and is extremely common in our pressure-filled society. People cannot slow down long enough to take care of their own bodies, and the resultant stress from a myriad of sources tears our bodies apart.

Combating stress requires an interdisciplinary approach involving biofeedback, psychotherapy, and physical-therapy techniques such as massage and relaxation exercises. Unfortunately, doctors just shrug off stress or offer the quick fix of a pill instead of offering constructive ways of coping with something that is pervasive in our society. Part of the problem is that doctors have a problem with trying to figure out how to deal with their own stress or just think of it as a fact of life.

Another example of the mind-body connection that doctors see daily in their offices is the "white-coat syndrome." I have a habit of not wearing a white coat most of the time because it feels too uncomfortable in the heat of Texas summers, and as I have grown older, I like being comfortable. I never thought it made me a better doctor, anyway.

My nurse always checks my patients' blood pressures when they come into the office. I have a habit of checking the blood pressure myself; it's one of my idiosyncrasies. I guess it's because I feel something is missing if I don't check it. Old habits die hard.

Over the past seventeen years, I have seen an interesting phenomenon. At least two-thirds of my patients have significantly higher blood pressures (twenty to thirty millimeters of mercury) when I check it compared to my nurse's readings. At first, I thought this was due to the aggravation of waiting, but it is independent of a time factor.

It also does not depend on how well the patient knows me. New or old, the patients just tend to run higher pressures when in my presence. It also does not depend on the sex of the patient. My eighty-year-olds react no differently than my forty-year-olds. I was actually starting to get a complex until I realized that this is a common problem that becomes a dilemma in patient management.

Blood pressure is not a static physiologic factor. It is labile in many people and changes with their state of mind. Things such as stress can increase blood pressure tremendously. Going to the doctor is an example of such a stress for many people.

The dilemma for a doctor is how to treat this problem. Usually, I try to have patients monitor their readings at home. Many people can't afford blood-pressure cuffs or don't feel comfortable taking their own readings.

If patients check their pressure at home and their readings are normal, I don't usually worry too much about "white-coat hypertension." Labile blood pressure is difficult to treat and is a big nemesis for both patient and doctor. My ego won't allow the thought that my presence is responsible for pushing my patients' blood pressures through the roof.

Without getting into the specifics of stress management, there are techniques that are useful to help cope with stress.

Both the doctor and the patient have to be willing to do more in treating the entire problem rather than just the symptoms. We all need to take control of our lives and sometimes change things that need to be changed, even if it is unpleasant. That involves lifestyle modification.

Helping people change their lifestyles is not easy and requires a holistic approach, not just focusing on a disease process or on "textbook medicine." Doctors have to go beneath the surface, and that requires concern and a precious commodity, time, that often are not reimbursed by insurance companies. Physicians first need to be willing to sacrifice their time in order to do the things that are important for their patients. This is both the right thing to do and part of practicing sound medicine. We can't let insurance companies dictate how we spend our time with our patients!

Unfortunately, a fact of life in our society is that doctors often spend the most time on the things for which they are well reimbursed and discard the rest as being too time consuming and unimportant. A lot of doctors feel that they cannot economically survive if they spend a lot of time just talking to their patients. The responsibility of educating patients often falls into the hands of the nurse and many times just gets ignored.

Both doctors and the insurance industry poorly understand the mind-body connection. Helping people to find ways to help themselves is important to their physical and mental well-being. Doctors need to be at the forefront of establishing a system that makes a high priority of the mind-body connection and that understands its value and importance in our healthcare structure. Our current system is only in its infancy in understanding how this connection works and in how our knowledge can be incorporated into traditional medical care. We just don't know all the answers, but what we are learning is intriguing!

The Importance of Self-Renewal

Stephen Covey defines four basic dimensions of renewal, and they are equally important for everyone to practice in their daily lives. They are: the physical, the mental, the social/emotional, and the spiritual.

As Covey states in *The 7 Habits of Highly Effective People*:

"The physical dimension involves caring effectively for our physical body—eating the right kinds of foods, getting sufficient rest and relaxation, and exercising on a regular basis."[2]

Covey could not have been more correct in his assessment of the importance of the physical realm in people's everyday lives. We are a product of both the abuse and the nurturing that we give our bodies. Doctors need to emphasize the importance of proper nutrition and exercise in preserving the greatest assets that we have—our physical beings.

A variety of studies have shown that exercise is important in preventing heart disease and a variety of illnesses.[3] Obesity is also an all too common precursor for other medical problems. It is important as well in psychological well-being because it helps to combat anxiety and depression. It is also an important tool in stress management. There is no doubt in my mind that people who exercise regularly as they get older stay physically younger and have an overall lower rate of physical disability.

The mental dimension of renewal involves refreshing our minds and keeping them active. A lot of us forget how to read after our formal education stops, and we watch an awful lot of television and play Nintendo, neither of which requires much thinking. Some of us use them as a diversion from thinking.

We need to continue to keep our minds active through reading, writing, or organizing and planning our lives. My patients who keep their minds active suffer less from depression and from memory loss. Keeping active is as important to us mentally as it is physically.

The spiritual realm of renewal is very individualized. For some it involves prayer; for some, meditation; and for some, a recommitment to what is important in their lives. As Covey so beautifully puts it:

> **"The spiritual dimension is your core, your center, your commitment to your value system. It's a very private area of life and a supremely important one. It draws upon the sources that inspire and uplift you and tie you to the timeless truths of all humanity."[4]**

We need to learn how to center ourselves and find inner peace in our lives. We need to draw upon our values and decide what our mission is in life. This requires setting priorities to spend time with prayer and meditation or whatever helps us to settle our inner conflicts and to find balance and peace in our lives. These beautiful words of Wendell Berry describe one man's ability to find peace.

The Peace of Wild Things

"When despair for the world grows in me
And I wake in the night at the least sound
In fear of what my life and my

children's lives may be,
I go and lie down where the wood drake
Rests in his beauty on the water,
and the great heron feeds,
I come into the peace of wild things
Who do not tax their lives with forethought
Of grief. I come into the presence of still water.
And I feel above me the day-blind stars
Waiting with their light. For a time
I rest in the grace of the world, and am free."

The final dimension involves the social and emotional aspects of our lives. It is important to keep the priorities in our relationships with others who are important in our lives. This involves a commitment to our families, to serving others in our community, and to being able to communicate with empathy to others.

Doctors need to realize the importance of renewal in their own lives as well as in the lives of those whom they try to heal. It is especially important to help deal with the daily stresses and burdens that are part of our daily lives. It is also critical to be able to find peace within ourselves so that we can help others find that peace. People often do not take the time to do what is important in their own lives, and doctors are no exception.

No one can cure the world with a pill or a simple pat on the shoulder. It is an understatement to say that life is far more complicated than that. Life gives us the opportunity to reach the finish line and be happy and content when we are done, but it takes hard work and setting priorities to reach life's goals.

Helping others gives life meaning. The words of George Bernard Shaw very aptly describe those whose lives gain meaning through service:

"This is the true joy in life—that being used for a purpose recognized by yourself as a mighty one. That being a force of nature, instead of a feverish, selfish little clod of ailments and grievances complaining that the world will not devote itself to making you happy. I am of the opinion that my life belongs to the whole community and as long as I live it is my privilege to do for it whatever I can. I want to be thoroughly used up when I die. For the harder I work the more I live. I rejoice in life for its own sake. Life is no brief candle to me. It's a sort of splendid torch which I've got to hold up for the moment and I want to make it burn as brightly as possible before handing it on to future generations."[5]

I will give of myself until my time on this earth is done, but life and death are not mine to give or to take. Remember that although I became a doctor, I was born a human being, and I am a child of God, no more and no less. When it comes time to pass the torch, I want to be remembered as a man who made mistakes but finished the race a better human being than when he started.

I want my family and friends to remember me as a compassionate man who tried his best to help others, but I also want my children to think of me as a father who tried his best to teach them what is important in life. After all, the legacy of a doctor is found in those whom he loves and in those who love him.

THE END

Endnotes

1. Larson and Koenig, "Is God Good for Your Health? The Role of Spirituality in Medical Care," *The Cleveland Clinic Journal of Medicine*, Vol. 67, No. 2, p. 80.
2. Covey, *The 7 Habits of Highly Effective People* (Simon and Schuster, 1989), p. 289.
3. Ibid., p. 290.
4. Ibid., p. 292.
5. George Bernard Shaw, Ibid., p. 299.

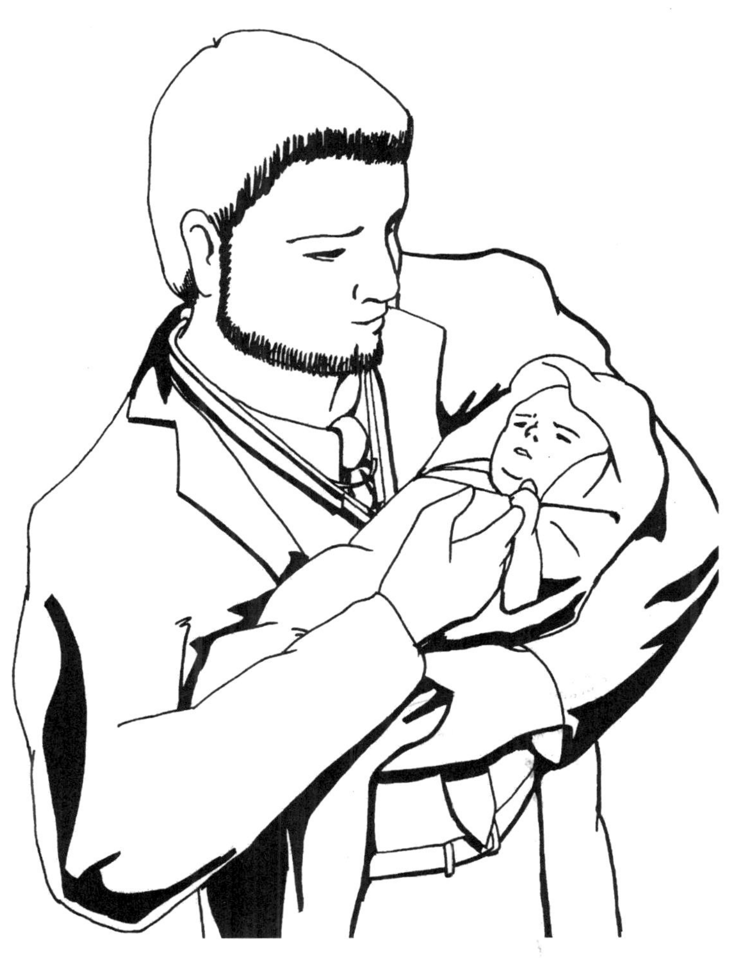

Afterthoughts

This book was stolen. It was stolen from a demanding medical practice that is a jealous mistress. I took notes in between patients, woke up thinking about it in the middle of the night, wrote during lunch hours, and daydreamed as I drove to and from work. My hat is off to all authors, especially to those who are doctors and still actively take care of patients. I realize how difficult creating a book really is, especially when you are new at it and you are already working ten to twelve hours a day.

For this book to be effective, I felt that it was necessary to bare my soul to my readers. My mission was to show you, through my experiences, a side of doctors that you may never have seen before. It was also important to show you a little about how the system works, with its strong points and weaknesses, while at the same time unveiling my own strengths and weaknesses. If I had been anything less than candid about myself, I would have sabotaged my own mission. And this book was a mission! Just ask my family and friends.

I wanted you to see that there is both a sad and a humorous side to being a doctor. The only way to accomplish this was to transport you into the world that I lived in for over twenty years of my life.

Our world has evolved and changed dramatically over that time, but certain values have not changed and hopefully will never be forgotten. No matter how society changes the rules of the game, we are all still human, and certain values are timeless. I wanted to share with you the values that my experience has taught me are the most important to both doctors and their patients.

I wrote this book with passion, the same passion that it took to get me through medical school, and the same burning desire that I feel every single day of my life as a doctor. If this book helps you to understand some of the agony and the ecstasy that I have felt during my career, my efforts will have been worthwhile.

This is the story about my journey, a journey that took me from confusion to a better understanding of why I am here on this earth. I am not claiming to have found the answers to the deepest secrets of life any more than I can claim to have found the fountain of youth. What I have learned is that peace and happiness can't be found in a textbook or by hiding behind a white coat or any other disguise, for that matter. Work offered me tempting illusions of peace and dangerous ways to cope with the pressures and pains of life.

God eventually brought me to my knees. There was nowhere else for me to go. My happiness was right in front of my face, but I was too blind to see it. I had to be ready to be the student instead of the teacher, a patient rather than a doctor. I had to understand and accept that I couldn't do it all by myself. I needed God's love and grace in order to heal myself, and I needed to find harmony in my professional, spiritual, and personal lives.

Life was never meant to be easy for any of us. I know that I am human and accept myself as less than perfect. No initials after my name could change the fact that I am vulnerable to life's pain, temptations, and suffering. I know that I can't finish the race by myself. Can you?

I am hoping that this book will prompt questions about the high rate of suicide, addiction, and divorce among doctors. Is there something that we are doing wrong in the screening process of medical school applicants? Should we provide more adequate psychological counseling for our medical students and young doctors? Is the almost inhuman pressure that we place upon our trainees allowing them to bend far enough to break?

Is it just too easy for doctors to get hold of drugs and find ways to self-destruct? Nothing prevents a doctor from prescribing most drugs either for himself or for his family. This practice has to stop and controls need to be put in place!

I hope that this book will allow the reader to see that while we are preparing good doctors, we are doing a poor job teaching them how to cope with living in the real world. We need to produce doctors that are not only book-smart but also street savvy. We need to educate our doctors about the "facts of life." That includes teaching them about managed care, educating them about the importance of economics, and giving them an understanding about the business end of running a medical practice.

Our system needs to teach doctors how to show compassion and at the same time not rob them of that compassion by being overly rigid and by ignoring their emotional needs. It is also time to teach our doctors how to take care of themselves physically and spiritually so that they can care for others more effectively.

We produce good doctors who often ignore their own problems and have no idea what they are getting into when they step outside of the ivory tower of medical school. Many are naïve and are taken advantage of by others who know that doctors are vulnerable prey.

It is important to raise questions about managed care, malpractice, and the cost of prescription drugs. These social issues affect doctors as well as their patients. I want to raise your level of awareness about these issues and raise questions about whether our current system is healthy for either our doctors or their patients.

Our system is broken and needs to be fixed. Unfortunately, many of our doctors find themselves in the same plight. Many of them are emotionally, physically, and spiritually bankrupt.

This book is meant to be thought provoking and at the same time playfully humorous. I wanted this book to capture the essence of what it is like to be a patient and a doctor in today's world. I hope that you can now sense that being a doctor is not just a combination of the "sublime and the ridiculous" but is primarily about compassion, love, and understanding.

About the Author

My first introduction to a stethoscope was in Elizabeth, New Jersey, on August 30, 1951. Approximately twenty-one years later, after attending Rutgers College and graduating Phi Beta Kappa with honors in English, I attended Hahnemann Medical College and Hospital in Philadelphia, Pennsylvania. I became a doctor in 1977 after graduating with honors in Pharmacology and Radiation Therapy. I was named to AOA (Alpha Omega Alpha), the national medical honor society.

My internship and residency training was at Baylor College of Medicine in Houston, Texas, where I also did my cardiology fellowship. After "serving my time," I went into private practice in Conroe, Texas, in 1983. I have been there ever since.

I am board certified in Internal Medicine and Cardiovascular Diseases and have twice been Chairman of the Department of Cardiology at Conroe Regional Medical Center. I am a Fellow of the American College of Cardiology and am proud to have performed the first heart catheterization in Montgomery County, Texas, in 1986.

I have published medical research in ***Seminars in Oncology***, ***Clinical Research***, and in ***Circulation***.

I have three sons and a wonderful family. Currently, I reside in The Woodlands, Texas.

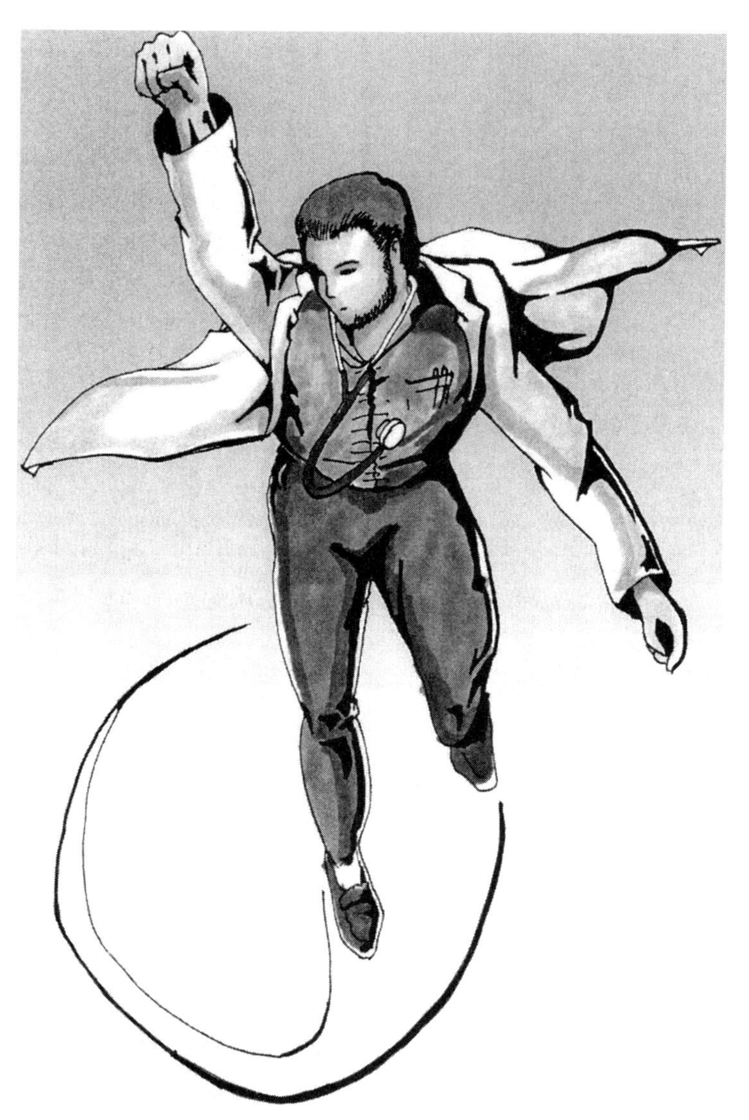

Index

C

D

E

F

G

H

I

J

K

L

M

N

O

P

W

X

Y